LIVING WITH THE DISABLED: YOU CAN HELP

A FAMILY GUIDE
BY JAN COOMBS

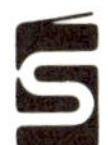
STERLING PUBLISHING CO., INC. NEW YORK
Distributed in the U.K. by Blandford Press

To Lisa, for her example of courage and patience

Edited and designed by Frederick Sard

Library of Congress Cataloging in Publication Data

Coombs, Jan.
    Living with the disabled.

    Bibliography: p.
    Includes index.
    1. Handicapped—Psychology.   2. Handicapped—
Family relationships.   3. Rehabilitation.   4. Handi-
capped—Services for.   I. Title.
RM930.C63   1984   362.4   83-24298
ISBN 0-8069-5578-3
ISBN 0-8069-7840-6 (pbk.)

CONTENTS

I WAS FORTUNATE ENOUGH TO HAVE HAD the opportunity to see this book evolve. Reading the manuscript as it progressed, I followed the author as she incorporated theory, research, personal experience and practical know-how into her work in order to facilitate an understanding from the family's perspective of the experience of severe illness or disability and, perhaps more important, how best to cope with it.

Rehabilitation is a process built around the physical, emotional and social problems of the disabled person and his family, in which the rehabilitation service attempts to solve these problems or at least bring about the best possible adjustment to them. However, all too often rehabilitation practitioners fail to appreciate and address family needs or recognize and utilize family strengths and resources in the rehabilitation "team" effort.

This book reflects in a very clearcut manner the need for active family involvement in the entire rehabilitation process. Practitioners must recognize the patient's family as a vital rehabilitative force, and the family must develop awareness of its potential for constructive participation.

The author has drawn on her own experience as a parent of a severely injured daughter. She has used this most effectively, as a catalyst for creating a book to assist others facing the challenge of disability or chronic illness in a family member. Basing her work on the premise that family involvement is crucial to rehabilitation success, the author explains how a knowledgeable, dedicated family can assist the patient to make best use of his residual capabilities, thereby increasing the potential for recovery.

A comprehensive and practical book for families of patients with a severe illness or disability has been needed for a long time. Families are often frightened by their emotional reactions to disability, unaware of their psychological needs and bewildered by the experiences of acute medical care, transition to and involvement in rehabilitation, and care following discharge, with its array of available resources. This book addresses these concerns, as well as many others, in a manner certain to help any family seeking information, advice and reassurance.

ROBERT D. MASON, Ph.D.
Rehabilitation Psychologist
Marshfield Clinic
Marshfield, Wis.

PREFACE

> As you wander on through life, brother,
> No matter what your goal,
> Keep your eye upon the doughnut
> And not upon the hole.
>
> Anonymous

As MY HUSBAND AND I WERE PREPARING for bed late on the evening of December 4, 1977, our telephone rang. The sound hardly registered in my mind: Nighttime phone calls are a normal part of life in my husband's profession. This call, like so many others, was from the hospital emergency room.

"Dr. Coombs here," said my husband as he shoved the receiver against his ear and automatically started to put his shoes back on.

"Yes ... Oh, no! Is she still alive?" he asked. "Yes ... I see ... Badly? Yes, we'll be right over!"

"*We'll* be right over?" I asked, puzzled. "Is it. . . ?"

Our eyes met, both of us remembering accident scenes in emergency rooms where we had worked, for me years ago, for him all too recently. Now one of ours, someone we loved, was hurt.

Soon afterwards, as we approached the hospital emergency entrance, we could hear our daughter Lisa's screams, mingled with the cries and groans of others. As we rushed through the door my husband gave my hand a tight squeeze, trying to give me the strength to face what we both knew awaited us.

During the next few hours the hospital staff—our friends and my

9

husband's co-workers—kept us from seeing Lisa. But we could still hear her cries as we conferred with the specialists who streamed in and out of her examining room. We learned that she had been involved in a head-on automobile collision. Her doctors thought she would live, and as far as they could determine, had suffered no brain damage. But her injuries were extensive and serious, and she would require immediate surgery. She had severe facial injuries, including multiple jaw fractures; she had lost most of her teeth, part of her tongue and parts of her upper and lower jawbones. In addition, her collarbone, left arm and left leg were broken and her right ankle crushed. The doctors could not rule out internal injuries, and were concerned that trauma to one of her breasts might require its eventual amputation.

It was noon the following day before we were finally permitted to see Lisa. She had just emerged from surgery. Nothing in our respective medical experiences had prepared us for the shock. There on the hospital bed, in place of our pretty eighteen-year-old daughter, was the body of a young girl whose only recognizable features were her eyes, eyes filled with fear, pain and bewilderment.

Her cleanshaven head was discolored and swollen to the size of a volleyball. A large metal frame, attached to her skull and lower jaw by long steel screws, encircled her head to stabilize what was left of her jaw. Her lips, once a pretty bow, were swollen and filled with black suture stitches.

As we neared her bed, she reached out for us with her free hand. Unable to speak, she pleaded with her eyes for help. Desperately trying to control our voices and expressions so as not to convey our fears, we tried ineptly to give her reassurance. After a few minutes, recognizing our distress and anxious to resume post-operative care, her nurses asked us to leave.

Looking back now, the months that followed seem like a nightmare. Interminable days of anxious waiting as Lisa lay in intensive care stretched out to weeks filled with constant visits to the hospital and then to long months of convalescence frequently interrupted by the need for more surgery. There were peaks of elation when Lisa surprised us all with her progress and valleys of dejection when complications arose. Imperceptibly we found ourselves discovering hitherto untapped strengths and developing new values as Lisa slowly continued to mend.

Two-and-a-half years after her accident, I was sitting across a table from Lisa at a restaurant in a nearby city to which she had recently moved. I was admiring her long, curly hair and sparkling eyes, unable to see her facial scars in the dimly lit room. Her left leg was propped up on a chair beside me, the ankle encased in yet another kind of steel frame. This one, having stabilizing pins running through her leg and foot, was the consequence of her fourteenth surgical procedure.

Lisa was telling me excitedly about her new life as a full-time civil engineering student at a technical school. She joked about her experiences trying to maneuver with her foot frame and crutches, and the complications this caused at school. I was still laughing about her latest escapade, a party she had given for her fellow classmates, when she suddenly became serious and said, "I've got something very important to tell you, Mom."

More than a little alarmed, I asked what it was.

"Oh, it's nothing *awful!*" she answered, spotting my worried frown. "I just wanted you to know that I've come to view my accident as a positive event in my life. Sure, I wish that it hadn't happened. But I realize all these experiences in the last few years have made me into a person I could never have become any other way. I'm proud of myself, I really appreciate my life, and I know I can handle anything else that happens to me."

I looked at the confident young woman sitting across from me and remembered the happy-go-lucky, undirected and unmotivated child of a few years before. Tears began to stream down my face, an outpouring of so many emotions ...

I am tempted to tell the whole story of my daughter's recovery—the remarkable transformation of her, at first uncertain in mind and mangled in body, into a self-assured woman who knows she can take on the world despite her residual handicaps. But that is not the purpose of this book. Proud as I am of Lisa's accomplishments, I have an even more important story to tell about the lessons we learned. Coming as we did from medical backgrounds, my husband and I knew a great deal about doctors, nurses, hospitals and health care services. Suddenly forced to be on the receiving end of these services, however, made us acutely aware of how much we didn't know and how difficult it can be to find needed resources. Our experiences made me realize that others with less knowledge of medical and rehabilitative services might have even more difficulty.

Each year in this country thousands of people are involved in accidents that leave them disabled. Countless others suffer from diseases that maim their bodies or otherwise restrict activity. Often these newly disabled people never get over their initial reaction to this unhappy turn of fate. They spend the rest of their days bitter and resentful, handicapped emotionally as well as physically.

Confronted with loss of a body part or function, many patients and their families and friends concentrate on the loss rather than on remaining abilities and resources. They tend to forget that everyone (even one who considers himself normal and healthy) has limitations, and that most of us, with our varying degrees of intelligence, talent and physical prowess, have learned to live within the limits of our capabilities.

Those of us who are closest to the patient are often in the best position to help, because we are the most concerned about his recovery and usually spend more time with him than anyone else does. Instead of standing on the sidelines helplessly wringing our hands, we can take an active role in helping the patient lead a useful, happy life. We can concentrate on what he has left, rather than what he has lost. With effort and determination, we can help him to "keep his eye upon the doughnut and not upon the hole."

In this book my primary emphasis is on the patient whose condition will respond to treatment, who can reasonably expect a degree of recovery. Readers who are concerned about someone whose prospects are less hopeful, particularly one whose death is imminent, may find that portions of this book are irrelevant to their needs or too optimistic for their circumstances. But the likelihood of death does not negate the importance of help. It only focusses that help on the more immediate goal of making each remaining day of the patient's life as full and satisfying as possible. To that end, readers with relatives or friends who are terminally ill will find much information here that is practical.

The desire to help a disabled person is not enough. We must know how to help and where to go for needed resources. This book, then, is for anyone close to someone who has had a traumatic accident or suffers from a debilitating disease—anyone who cares and wants to know how to help.

ALTHOUGH THE IDEA FOR THIS BOOK came out of my family's experiences and what we learned, I could not have completed this work without the help of many other people. I thank those disabled individuals and their families who told me their experiences that others might learn from them. Brief episodes from these case histories illustrate the text, with fictitious names given (except for references to my daughter Lisa). I thank also the many health care professionals, working with disabled people, without whose encouragement this entire project would have been impossible. Their guidance through three years of research gave me the material I wanted to include in this book. Those who answered my requests for information, granted me interviews, gave me advice or read my various drafts include Jeanne Batten, Elva Bennett, Ron Braun, Michael Brooks, Pat Buehler, Jim Hansen, Dory Holmes, Jim Jewell, Gil Johnsson, Sheldon Kaye, Kenneth Kolpan, Anthony Magliozzi, Carl Meissner, Peter Mick, Mark Moser, Nancy Jo Patterson, Lori Pederson, Margaret Peterson, Peter Quinn, Jessica Robbins-Miller, John Roehmer, Charles Sabatier, Jr., Dale Sternberg, Leonard Shubetowski, Dale Trimberger, Dick Williams, Alana Ziaya and Al Zimmerman.

Most especially, I thank Bob Mason for his unflagging interest and assistance during the four-year course of this project. His suggestions and critical reviews of my drafts were vital to many parts of this book.

I am also indebted to Fred Sard, my editor at Sterling, for his scrupulous attention to detail and kind suggestions that helped to hone this book to its final, far more readable, form.

Although I gratefully acknowledge all the help these people have given me, I assume full responsibility for any errors or omissions found herein.

Finally, and most of all, I thank my husband, children and friends for their wholehearted support and encouragement during this book's lengthy gestation, and my mother-in-law for her tireless search through my many drafts for typing errors.

CHAPTER 1

"This Couldn't Happen to Me!": Adjusting to Disability

WHEN SOMEONE WE KNOW AND LOVE becomes disabled, there is no comfort in numbers. Over 1,000 Americans are severely hurt in accidents every hour, leaving a yearly toll of about 350,000 victims with permanent impairments, but the fact that so many others are injured does nothing to lessen our grief. Nor does it help us to know that 22 million Americans—one out of every six adults between the ages of eighteen and sixty-four—are disabled due to accident or chronic ill-health.[1]

Conditioned as we are today by all the news about medical advances, we have come to expect long and healthy lives. We place excessive importance on athletic prowess and sound, beautiful bodies, and tend to avoid those who are less than perfect, with disabilities that disfigure or impair normal functioning. We disregard statistics about accidents and potentially crippling diseases. We view good health and soundness of mind and body not just as desirable goals but as inalienable rights.

Thus, when a family member or close friend becomes seriously ill or injured, we are stunned. Suddenly the life shared with that person is transformed. The building blocks of our security tumble in disarray. Perhaps a husband loses his ability to earn a living or a wife her ability to care for her family. An aging parent who has always enjoyed self-reliance—or a grandchild who has recently attained it—may become dependent on us for care. Or a friend who has given special meaning to our lives can no longer share in our activities.

Facing the possibility that a loved one may die, we are tortured by fears of loss, by uncertainty and despair. If the danger of death recedes, the character of our misery changes. We begin to fear that his life will be filled with seemingly endless pain and sorrow. While it is a relief to learn that he will live, we worry that he will continually suffer.

Inevitably in such circumstances we want to help, to somehow remove the cause of suffering or at least relieve the pain and anxiety. But all too often, we feel helpless.

Most of us do some things automatically when friends or relatives are ill. We run errands, help with the care of young children or aged parents and prepare meals. We try to ensure that the patient receives the best available care. We visit and send flowers and cards to express concern. Yet somehow there is a desire to do more.

Although we can help a disabled person in countless ways, we cannot assume that everything we do to help will be beneficial. Well-intentioned efforts can cause great harm if, for example, too much is done at the wrong time. Wanting to help is not enough, then. Knowing how and when to help is crucial.

Beyond mere practical favors, expressions of concern and assurances of competent care, we can do much more. All of these activities should, to a greater or lesser degree, involve the giving of emotional support that will help the patient adjust to his disability. This kind of help can be the greatest gift. It is one that a person who loves and cares is well qualified to give.

To help the patient in this most meaningful way, however, we need to know something about attitudes and emotional reactions to disability. And we need to understand how patients learn to adjust to disability, so we can constructively participate in this process.

ATTITUDES TOWARDS DISABILITY

Attitudes towards disability are not predictable because they depend upon personal experience and environment. Each of us reacts quite differently to our own or another's injury or illness.

The severity of a disability matters less than how we think it will affect our lives—the degree to which it threatens our goals and security. Most of us would probably consider the loss of a little finger to be of relatively small consequence, but such an injury can spell the end of a career for a professional musician. One woman who loses a breast is grateful for the surgery because her doctor is confident of a cancer cure; another wants to die because she can't tolerate the idea that she is disfigured and sexually unattractive. The amputation of a leg has far different meanings for an eighty-year-old diabetic and an eighteen-year-old athlete. And an elderly amputee who was already living with his family may suffer less of a loss than one who loses his leg and the ability to live independently both in one blow.

Sometimes bystanders suffer more disruption in their lives than the patient. A woman who is forced to give up a promising career to care for an invalid relative may find her life intolerably disrupted, while her relative is delighted to have the additional attention. A man who can no longer finance his children's education, because his mother requires nursing-home care after a stroke, may be sorely disturbed, while his mother, although in drastically altered circumstances, is hardly aware of her condition or its consequences.

An individual's personality, past history of success and failure and methods of coping with stress all influence his reactions to disability. A basically optimistic, assertive and independent person is more likely to view the disability as a new challenge. But one who thinks of life as a never-ending succession of uncontrollable disappointments will tend to feel victimized, dependent and hopeless.

Then, too, the nature of the onset and course of the disability plays a part in shaping attitudes. Sometimes the emotional impact of sudden crippling from an accident is far greater for the patient and those close to him than a situation in which everyone has months or years to prepare for total disablement. On the other hand, someone with a progressively deteriorating disability may experience more fear in contemplating future loss of body function than one forced to confront immediate loss.

Research on attitudes towards disability among the general population shows that some forms of disability are thought more shameful than others.[2] Conditions that disfigure the body or affect the mind, for example, are usually considered more shameful than those that are invisible or leave the mind intact. (However, even though visible forms of disability are considered less desirable, many disabled people wish their infirmities were more obvious so that others' attitudes would be more appropriate; for example, patients with arthritis or heart disease often complain that their families or co-workers do not understand why they cannot perform certain tasks.)

Our prejudices about disability influence our overall perspective. If we think of disabled people only as helpless objects of pity, our reaction when disability strikes close to home will undoubtedly be gloomy. On the other hand, if we view disabled people as individuals capable of being independent and productive, our outlook will be far more optimistic.

Finally, the prospects for rehabilitation can affect attitudes towards disability. When we see a possibility of improvement, we respond differently from when we are convinced that recovery is impossible.

Everyone involved in a disability, then—whether as patient, relative or friend—views the condition with a different set of attitudes. We must acknowledge these underlying attitudinal differences in order to appreciate the wide variety of emotional reactions to disability.

EMOTIONAL REACTIONS TO
THE ONSET OF DISABILITY

These emotional reactions are the same as those commonly experienced with any form of loss, whether the death of a spouse, loss of a job or dissolution of a marriage. Whatever the loss, a variety of feelings are experienced that are distressing to the deprived and to everyone around him. These emotional reactions to loss are unconscious defenses to protect the conscious mind from situations too painful to face directly. They are essential to the emotional healing process each of us must go through in adjusting to new circumstances in life.

We need to understand these responses for two reasons First, because we experience these feelings ourselves when someone close to us becomes disabled. If we realize they will pass in time, we may find them more tolerable. Second, we can better recognize these feelings in the patient, accept them as normal responses and help him begin the emotional healing process—the process of adjustment to disability.

These reactions to loss, disability and death have been described by many professionals. Dr. Nancy Kerr has examined these reactions from the patient's perspective.[3] Her description of this process can also be applied to those at the bedside, who share the loss and disruption in their lives.

Dr. Kerr defines the first reaction to disability as one of shock and denial: "This couldn't happen to me!" If the patient is not so drugged or dazed that he is unaware of his physical condition, he may still shut out all that has happened, rejecting the evidence of his senses because it does not fit his image of himself as a whole and healthy person.

Upon first hearing that someone we love has had an accident or suffers from a serious disease, we are stunned. Then we begin to look for an explanation to show that what we have heard is untrue: "Perhaps they have the wrong person in the emergency room," "Possibly the doctor has made the wrong diagnosis," "Maybe I didn't hear correctly," "Nothing this bad could happen to someone I love," we reason in our dazed condition.

Confronted by all the evidence of his disability, the patient finally admits his condition but decides to overcome it: "I'm sick, but I'll get well. And I'll do anything to recover." While this attitude seems admirable on the surface, its foundations are weak. The patient is saying that if only he works hard enough he will no longer have the disability; then he will be the same as before. In this emotional state he will do anything to overcome his new condition, but he will not try anything that might help him learn to function with it.

And we who stand by offer optimistic platitudes: "Don't worry, you'll be as good as new in no time," we say, being equally capable of false hope as we live through our grief.

As the patient contemplates his loss and finds he can no longer do things he was used to doing, little cracks appear in his fortress of emotional defenses. He thinks about his destroyed goals and concludes that his disability has ruined his life, that all is lost. He says, "This is it. I'm never going to be like I was before." He is consumed by self-pity and regards himself as inadequate and worthless. He becomes angry with everyone, including himself. He mourns for the way of life he has lost.

In our grief for our disabled relative, we search for explanations and try to place blame. We become angry and frustrated. We direct our hostility towards others—friends, relatives, employers, doctors, nurses—towards ourselves, towards God. We wonder what we could have done differently or did not do. We feel guilty and depressed.

Others who have studied emotional reactions to disability contend that these feelings may occur in a different order or that other feelings may occur. Be that as it may, the important point here is that shock, denial, self-pity, anger, guilt and depression are all normal feelings regardless of the sequence in which they take place. The patient and those close to him may experience extremely painful feelings, but these are necessary steps in the healing process.

PERSONAL DIFFERENCES IN
ADJUSTING TO DISABILITY

Everyone adjusts to disability at a different speed. While the patient is in one particular emotional state, those around him are struggling with another. This situation can lead to unpredictable behavior and many misunderstandings. For example, the patient may refuse to see visitors one day, yet make impossible demands the next. A husband may reject his wife's expressions of love because he blames the whole world for his disability, but she interprets his behavior as a personal rejection. Conversely, she may suddenly blame him for his illness, because she is trying to find some reason for this unhappy disruption in their lives. At home, meanwhile, family members feel neglected because of the attention focussed on the patient and begin to fight with one another just when their cooperation is most needed.

Just as some people take longer to heal their physical wounds, some need more time to heal emotional wounds. An individual's general emotional health and the kinds of support he gets from those around him influence the speed at which he heals. Although some people adjust to disability within a few weeks or months, others take years and, sadly, some never adjust. The same can be said for friends and relatives—some never adjust to the disability of a loved one.

Regardless of the severity of an injury or disease, the patient who no longer can perform activities he considers important takes longer to adjust. The musician who loses a finger, career and status all at once is apt to have much more difficulty than a mother who loses an arm but can still care for her children.

More critically, however, the patient's progress towards full adjustment will depend upon his ability to cope with stress. If he has always reacted to stress by running away and is now confined to bed, he will have to learn new ways to cope with the stress of his disability. Patients with limited experience and emotional resources, those who have resorted to unhealthy and ineffective methods of coping—such as denial, alcohol, other drugs, anger as a response to difficulty—are poorly equipped to handle the emotional problems of disability. They may require professional counselling. Those who are flexible and able to compromise and have a variety of healthy responses to stress can use some or all of them to overcome this new crisis in their lives.

Certain kinds of disabilities almost always seem to require a long adjustment time. Patients with spinal cord injuries, for example, often take two or more years to come to terms with their condition. Persons with progressively deteriorating neurological diseases or head injuries often require much longer periods of adjustment, as do their families.

Friends and relatives may find that they progress towards adjustment more rapidly than the patient. They generally suffer less disruption in their daily lives and have more time to think. A young wife who spends countless days at her husband's bedside, while waiting for him to regain consciousness after an accident, has ample time to review their life together and their plans, look at options and work through some of her feelings. While the patient's mind, inactivated by shock, anesthesia or drugs, is in a holding pattern, that of a spouse or friend is fully conscious and forced to think overtime, juggling what he sees and hears but may not want to know.

Conversely, a patient who must wait days or weeks for laboratory reports or spend long, empty hours in bed may have plenty of time to contemplate his life, losses and future, while his family, suddenly burdened with new responsibilities, has little time to think.

Clearly, the time needed to adjust to disability varies greatly with each individual. However long the process takes, we can help ensure that adjustment will eventually occur. There are many ways to do this, but the basis of all our activities should be the emotional support we can give. Subsequent chapters will examine how to help the patient at specific stages of treatment and recovery. Here we will now look in a more general way at suggestions for helping the patient as he moves from one emotional state to another, regardless of where he is in the treatment program.

Ways to Help With the Adjustment Process

At the time of the accident or discovery of illness, when the patient is in emotional or physical shock, or denying his condition, we need to recognize that this behavior is protecting him. Were he facing the full impact of his disability, he would feel extremely anxious and helpless. Instead of forcing him to do this, we should give him time to slowly get used to his condition. Initially, what he needs most is our comforting love—a hand to hold, given by someone willing to listen and say little.

> When Mrs. Parker emerged from anesthesia, she discovered that the doctor had performed a colostomy, creating an artificial opening for her bowel on her abdomen. She did not care to know that a malignancy had been removed or that people with colostomies lead normal lives. She was grappling with the image of the oozing hole on her abdomen, and wondering how anyone could love her. More than anything else right then, she needed the assurance of her husband's love.

On the other hand, although the patient does not want to know all about the condition at this point, great harm is done if we help in the denial of disability. We should try to answer questions truthfully and simply, without giving information the patient is not yet ready to accept.

Part of our task is to suggest to others how they can help the patient. We can explain to other family members and friends that in the beginning he is struggling to confront his disability. He cannot handle their questions or advice, but does need their comfort and support. Those who want to help should be encouraged to do so in appropriate ways, but discouraged from asking too many questions or sharing their experiences and advice with the patient.

Slowly the patient begins to realize what has happened to his body. He asks questions about treatment and possibilities for cure. He may decide that he can overcome his disability and be as he was before if he works hard enough. Even though this desire to cooperate in a treatment program is based on false hope at this point, his incentive can be channelled into useful activities.

A young quadriplegic, Tim Caywood, tells of his own experience: "If doctors and nurses had told me I would never walk again in the beginning, I would have given up altogether. A patient in the early stage should not be told anything that will take away any hope he may have."[4] Caywood's doctors had been unable to predict the full extent of his injuries, but they used his hope constructively without deceiving him with false hope. They used his willingness to cooperate in treatment to his ultimate advantage. Even though Caywood has never walked again, he has gained enough emotional strength to finally adjust to his injury. "Hope," he says, "is a very important defense weapon. Don't let anyone destroy it."

On the other hand, we need to guard against false hope—the sort that leads a patient from doctor to doctor, searching for a miracle cure.

Disability of any kind damages the image the patient has of himself. When he becomes disfigured or loses some abilities, he loses self-esteem. He begins to feel ugly, sexually unattractive and worthless. To improve his chances of recovery, his confidence must be restored. Even when he is motivated by unrealistic goals to cooperate in his treatment program, we can use his accomplishments during treatment to rebuild his self-confidence. As he begins to feel better about himself with each success, he will acquire the courage to tackle more difficult tasks and to finally come to terms with his disability.

Sincere praise is one of the best tools for restoring self-confidence, so we need to look for things to praise. We will need to look very carefully for small improvements and accomplishments— things we might otherwise take for granted—which show that the patient is trying to get better. Here we can make a significant contribution, having a distinct advantage over his doctors and nurses, because we have only one patient to observe.

As the patient starts to regain a lost skill or perform some simple task once more, we should be ready with praise. Quiet praise to the patient alone is not enough; we should proudly point out the accomplishment to other visitors and hospital staff. We might say, "Doesn't Mary's hair look nice? She was able to comb it herself today," or, "Dan sat up by himself for the first time this morning. Did you ever see such determination?"

Soon everyone around the patient is reinforcing our praise and offering their own encouragement. Because we are interested and have looked for small improvements, we have created an atmosphere in which the patient can begin to feel good about himself again.

Despite our best efforts, however, the day comes when the patient is in despair. As much as he is trying, he finally realizes he is never going to recover completely and function as before. For a long time he has been thinking, amidst all his hopes, about all the things he is unable to do. Gradually these thoughts have grown into a mountainous obstruction blocking his view of the future. Concluding he has nothing to live for, he gives up.

It is painful to see someone we love in mourning. We may be consumed with pity, perhaps because we share his feeling that his life holds no future, and we are as fearful and sad as he. Or we may be uncomfortable with his expressions of grief, his outbursts of crying, because we are repelled by such displays of emotion. However, the patient should be encouraged to express his feelings, because this period of mourning is an essential part of the healing process.

John Schatzlein, now Home Work Administrator and Counsellor for Control Data Corporation in Minneapolis, was a vigorous teen-age athlete when he damaged his spinal cord and had to learn to live in a wheelchair. Today he spends much of his time travelling around the country conducting workshops on sexual concerns of disabled people. Schatzlein says, "It's important for anyone who wants to help a disabled person to provide an atmosphere of trust and give that person all the time he needs to work through his feelings, to cry and to grieve. You can't rush the grief process."

The patient in mourning is immersed in comparisons—the way he is now versus the way he used to be, his loss of abilities versus the abilities of people who are whole and well. All he can see is his deficiencies. We should not try to stop his mourning, but instead respect his need to grieve, encourage the expression of his feelings and try to be understanding listeners. Perhaps we can do even more at this stage: While the patient is contemplating his losses, we can gently begin to show him what he has left.

Too often we tend to concentrate on disabilities rather than abilities. When we see someone in a wheelchair, our attention is focussed on the chair. We assume that whoever sits in that chair must be disabled in all respects, that he is *disabled as a person*. He is not. He is an individual who, although unable to do certain things, still possesses many skills and retains the basic qualities of his personality. In fact, he is apt to possess abilities that we lack.

Instead of focussing on losses then, we should look on the positive side. The patient knows what he has lost; we must use our energy and creativity to point out his remaining abilities.

Sometimes it helps to show the patient examples of people in similar situations who have come to terms with their disabilities and are leading fulfilling lives. This evidence makes him realize that his limitations need not cancel all rewarding activity.

> Bill, a young man with newly diagnosed diabetes, felt his life was now worthless because he thought he could no longer participate in sports. His mother discussed his depression with a friend, a woman he much admired. The next day this woman visited Bill in the hospital and casually mentioned her own diabetes.
>
> "You don't have diabetes!" said Bill. "I've seen the way you are on backpacking trips—you're active and healthy."

"Sure I have diabetes, Bill; it's a nuisance sometimes, what with all the fuss about diet and insulin shots, but I don't ever let it get in my way."

That short conversation was the turning point for Bill. When he realized that he could lead a normal life, he became motivated to learn how to control his disease rather than let it control him.

Such examples of others overcoming disability can be encouraging. However, they can also have the opposite effect. One paraplegic patient may see a story about someone in a wheelchair and think, "Great. She's getting around." But another may think, "Is that all I have to look forward to?" Those who know the patient well must use their judgment regarding his responses to such examples.

Well-chosen examples and comments can often help to resolve a patient's feelings about his disability, but sometimes remarks by well-intentioned visitors can destroy all his progress. Their comments are usually prompted by their discomfort in the sickroom. They do not know what to say, so they say something obvious—something that usually pertains to the patient's losses: "You're not going to be able to work at the shop anymore, are you, Joe? What are you going to do for a living?"

In this case, Joe's friends should be intercepted before they have a chance to see him, and informed that he is very worried about his job and income. They should be made to realize that they can help by thinking of ways for him to use his talents and remaining abilities: "Say, Joe, you've always been interested in electronics. Perhaps when you recover from your injuries you could enroll at West Tech. They do a good job of placing their graduates." While acknowledging his loss, Joe's friends should try to give him some positive things to think about.

Family members should take an active role, then, in suggesting ways in which other family members and friends can help. Confiding in them and enlisting their support encourages their constructive participation in the patient's recovery. Chances are good that they will be flattered and grateful to learn that they can help in very important ways.

In his own time, days, weeks or months later, the patient gradually comes to realize that his disability is part of his life, something that should not have happened but did. This realization gives him a solid foundation for adjustment to disability. He begins to develop new goals and values, to focus his energies towards new achievements. He learns to accept his limitations as he prepares to make the best possible use of his remaining abilities.

As Glorya Hale says in her *Source Book for the Disabled*, "Sometimes a person's view of his or her disability is more handicapping than the disability itself—some with severe disability and physical limitations don't view themselves as handicapped, while others whose disabilities are minor think of themselves as severely handicapped."[5] For our purposes, there is a difference between being handicapped and disabled, and that difference is one of attitude. Anyone with an injury or disease is disabled; however, not everyone with a disability is handicapped. The handicapping comes from the attitudes of the patient and those around him who think he is no longer capable of leading a useful life.

Helping a disabled person achieve a positive attitude about his life can be an arduous task, but it is a work of love. To that love, we might add the gift of humor.

Editor, author and lecturer Norman Cousins promotes the benefits of laughter in his book, *Anatomy of an Illness*, where he describes his battle and final victory over a crippling arthritic condition. Cousins was familiar with well-documented research on depression and other negative emotions as causative factors in disease. He reasoned that other, less well recognized theories about using positive thinking and humor to promote wellness could assist in his recovery. Using large doses of Allen Funt's *Candid Camera* television tapes and old Marx Brothers movies, he found that hearty belly laughter gave him more relief from pain and a greater sense of well-being than the pills he had previously taken. Laughter, Cousins concludes, *is* the best medicine.

In a recent interview, Cousins has said,

> Illness is not a laughing matter. Maybe it ought to be. Laughter is a form of internal jogging. It moves the internal organs around. It enhances respiration. It is an igniter of great expectations. Your body will experience a powerful gravitational pull in the direction of those expectations.

Pointing out that sad and angry emotions can cause illness, Cousins says,

> Incongruous though it may sound, if you have the capacity for joy, this will be the time to put it to fullest use. It makes no sense to believe that emotions have an effect on the body's chemistry only when they're on the downside.[6]

So we should tuck away our sad faces and bring out our smiles, looking for humor where we least expect to find it. When we help the patient to laugh, we infect him with a joy for living and a desire to recover.

For the patient to adjust to his disability he must first acknowledge that he is disabled. He must learn that his limitation may restrict and inconvenience him but does not devalue him as a person. If need be, he must acquire new goals for his life. Finally, he must develop new skills and enhance his remaining ones.

If the patient fails to adjust, he will continue to deny his disability, adhere to old values and goals that no longer apply and refuse to learn new skills. Constantly frustrated by his inability to live up to his former expectations, he will develop unsuccessful and even injurious ways of coping with his condition. He will never overcome his mourning or anger, and may resort to drugs or alcohol or withdraw into a protective shell from which he can only be rescued by professional counselling.

But it doesn't have to be that way. If we care, and if we help, we can make the difference.

CHAPTER 2

The Ins and Outs of Hospitals

A DISABLED PERSON IS LIKELY TO SPEND some time in a hospital at first—perhaps only a few days while doctors study his newly diagnosed disease and stabilize his condition, or possibly several weeks or months if he has been injured in a serious accident. Although hospitals are obvious places to go for treatment, they can be very frightening places for both patient and visitor. In that unfamiliar environment, where workers speak a strange language and practise unusual customs, even a harmless notice can be frightening.

Mrs. Snyder had just been admitted to the hospital for tests when a nurse posted an "NPO" sign over her bed. Shortly, the three other women in her room were given their meal trays.

"Can't my wife get anything to eat?" asked her husband.

"Of course not," answered the aide. "She's NPO."

Bewildered by that reply, Mr. and Mrs. Snyder waited for a while to ask the nurse what it meant, fearful of what she would tell them. When they finally gathered enough courage to ask, the nurse replied, "Oh, that's just a standard Latin abbreviation for 'nothing by mouth.' You can't have anything to eat or drink until after some of your tests."

In the hospital environment, there are few familiar procedures or items of equipment for the patient and his family. Anything can cause fear. When the patient is seriously ill and surrounded by strange equipment, these fears can reach gigantic proportions.[1]

Any form of illness, even a common cold, causes feelings of dependence in a patient. When he must rely on strangers for his care and does not understand what they are doing, he quickly feels that he has lost control of his body and life.

If the patient is to recover successfully he must feel in control and able to make important decisions about his treatment program. Patients who take no part in decisions about their care feel less need to comply with treatment orders and tolerate painful procedures poorly. If they agree only passively and reluctantly to a treatment program designed by other people, their chances for recovery are seriously threatened.[2]

While the patient is hospitalized, then, one of our tasks is to help him learn what is happening so that he can feel in control and participate intelligently in treatment decisions. In the words of psychologist Lee Meyerson, "The ideal helpers are like blockers on a football team—they run interference, clear paths, create opportunities and make it as easy as possible for the patient to take the ball and run with it. It's the patient's ball game."[3] "Running interference" for a patient is difficult when we know little about the playing field, the other players or the rules of the game. This chapter, then, contains information about hospitals and suggests ways to create opportunities for the patient. Finally, it examines discharge planning, a process that prepares him to leave the hospital.

FIRST DECISIONS

Choosing a Hospital

The kind and quality of care a hospital provides significantly influences a patient's chance for successful recovery. Since some hospitals are better than others, we ought to know how to evaluate them. Some patients never get to choose their hospital; they may be rushed to the facility nearest the scene of the accident, or their community may have only one hospital. But if the patient has the luxury of choice, and questions the care he is receiving in a particular hospital, he can use certain evaluation guidelines to judge its facilities and service.[4]

In general, large hospitals are preferable to smaller ones because they have a greater variety of treatment facilities and services. Many large hospitals, for example, have extensive rehabilitation programs in addition to their acute-care services. Association with a university medical school or postgraduate program is another good sign; such hospitals tend to provide a high level of care. Proprietary hospitals tend to be smaller and less well equipped; they often offer a minimum of services.

The Joint Commission on Accreditation of Hospitals has adopted stringent standards for reviewing hospital services and patient care. Those hospitals with accreditation are apt to provide better care than the 20 percent that either have failed to meet commission standards or have never applied for accreditation. Hospitals with accreditation display their documents for public inspection.

In large cities, a physician may be associated with several hospitals. The patient can ask his doctor about the advantages and disadvantages of each institution before they make a choice. Patients who live in an area having only one hospital—often a small one—must weigh the convenience of a local facility and care by a trusted physician against the advantages of care in a larger but distant hospital.

Choosing a Physician

Like hospitals, some physicians are better qualified than others. Many physicians have American Board of Medical Specialties certification, signifying expertise in a particular field of medicine— family practice, orthopedics, or physical medicine and rehabilitation, for example. Such certification does not guarantee excellence, but it can be a valuable tool for judging a physician's ability. Most state and county medical societies supply information about certified physicians who are licensed to practise in their area. Highly specialized physicians are often found at large medical institutions.

Beyond a doctor's diplomas, certificates and reputation, and every bit as important, is his ability to communicate with the patient—and with family members when they are trying to help the patient understand what is happening. If the physician is inaccessible, unapproachable or reluctant to answer questions about diagnosis and treatment in understandable terms, the patient will suffer from this failure in communication.

Many of us feel intimidated by doctors and are reluctant to take time from their busy schedules to ask for explanations. Usually, however, the best doctors—often the busiest—make time to answer questions. A good doctor will enter an examining room with no indication of rush; give full explanations, draw diagrams if need be and ask if the patient understands; give reasons for tests, treatments and medications; tell the patient what to expect and what he hopes to achieve; and leave instructions for reaching him, encouraging calls whenever a problem arises. The patient who has such a doctor is fortunate.

Most people have a regular physician to whom they turn for medical help; when their condition is serious enough to warrant consultation with a specialist, they can rely on their doctor to refer them to one who is well qualified. When someone must find a specialist on his own, he can contact a nearby university medical center or ask a local medical society for a list of physicians. Before making an appointment, he can telephone the doctor to discuss his problem. Frequently this brief conversation will give important clues about how he will relate to the physician in treatment.

Upon admission to a hospital that has a university teaching program, a patient may be offered a choice of private or "teaching service" ("ward") care. These designations refer to type of care received rather than room assignment. "Teaching service" care is administered by medical students or postgraduate residents under an "attending physician's" supervision. Some patients with sufficient financial resources refuse teaching service care because they do not want to be "bothered" by students. However, the quality of care on a teaching service is usually equal to private physician care. The attending physicians are usually specialty-board (A.B.M.S.) certified and are well informed about recent advances in their field, sharing their knowledge with the students, all to the patient's ultimate advantage. Being monitored by an expert often outweighs the inconvenience of having students involved in treatment.

Finding Answers and Help in the Hospital

Many different people are responsible for the patient's care in the hospital, and it is often difficult to know where to turn for help with a specific problem. Although one doctor is ultimately responsible for the treatment program, a patient may have many doctors. The attending physician or private doctor may call upon consultants, specialists with expertise in other areas of medicine. An accident victim, for example, may have consulting orthopedic, plastic and neurosurgeons, as well as cardiac and pulmonary specialists. These consultants are each involved in only one particular aspect of his care. The patient's family can discuss some parts of his treatment with each consultant, but need to know who is responsible for total care when they need information about his general condition or clarification of conflicting answers from the other doctors.

Nurses form the next line of command. Here again many nurses care for a single patient, changing bandages, administering medicines and checking equipment and his condition. Each change of shift brings a bewildering array of new personnel—nurses, nurse's aides and perhaps students. All these people can give help of a general nature, but some do not have the authority or knowledge to answer specific questions about the patient's condition or treatment. For this kind of information it is necessary to find out who is in charge of the patient on each particular shift.

Conscientious nurses consider teaching to be an important part of their duties. They explain the reasons for medications, tests and procedures, and interpret hospital regulations and doctor's orders. They welcome questions because they realize that understanding of treatment procedures will help the patient. Although we may be reluctant to display ignorance, we should not be afraid to ask questions.

Besides the nurses, a vast army of other hospital personnel— x-ray and laboratory technicians, orderlies, housekeepers, social workers, clergy—come to the patient's bedside with specific tasks to perform. All these people should be wearing name tags or some other indication of their staff position, and can be consulted at appropriate times for information or assistance.

Patients' Rights

Contrary to popular belief, patients do not have to shed their rights along with their clothes when they enter the hospital. In 1973 the American Hospital Association adopted a Patient's Bill of Rights to be used as a model by its members.[5] Although compliance is voluntary, the tenets of this declaration are based on sound legal precedent. In effect, health care institutions are expected to recognize and uphold these rights even if they have not formally adopted them. Most facilities provide newly admitted patients with material explaining the substance of these rights. The failure to do so may suggest a lack of concern for the patient; it does not relieve the hospital of its legal obligations to the patient. These rights include the following:

- the right to considerate and respectful care
- the right to know about diagnosis, treatment and chances of recovery, unless medically inadvisable, in which case this information will be given to an appropriate person on patient's behalf
- the right to understand and give informed consent to all treatments and procedures (except in emergencies), to be informed of medical risks and alternative courses of treatment and to know who will perform procedures
- the right to refuse treatment to the extent permitted by law and to be informed of the consequences of that action
- the right to privacy regarding patient's person and medical care
- the right to confidential medical records and to information regarding how records are used and who sees them
- the right to be advised of any aspects of care that are considered experimental or part of a research program, and the right to refuse to participate in such a project
- the right to reasonable continuity of care, including provisions for care after hospital discharge
- the right to examine and receive an explanation of the hospital bill regardless of source of payment
- the right to know what hospital rules and regulations apply to patient's conduct

Even in the best hospitals there are occasional incidents of negligence because staff is tired, overworked or momentarily inattentive. If we have complaints about care or suspicions that the patient's rights have been violated, we should discuss these concerns with the head nurse or doctor. Often a brief conversation will solve the problem.

> Mr. Dawson's family discovered that their hospitalized father was often put under restraint in bed at night. They talked with the head nurse and learned that elderly patients, who may have little difficulty at home, sometimes become confused in unfamiliar surroundings. Since Mr. Dawson had tried to get out of bed on several occasions, each time seriously disrupting his treatment

equipment and threatening his own safety, his night nurses obtained permission to apply restraints when he became confused.

Even though his family then understood the reason for the restraints, they were still concerned about their use. With the cooperation of the nursing staff, they arranged to stay with him during the night so he would no longer need the restraints.

If our questions are not so easily resolved, we can talk with someone in the hospital administration—a patient counsellor, ombudsman or advocate—who handles patient and family grievances. Questions or complaints about physician conduct are best directed to the chief of staff, the doctor responsible for handling problems relating to the performance of his colleagues in that institution.

Complaints about possible negligence are disagreeable to staff, particularly when they involve a co-worker or close friend. For this reason, a written complaint should be as factual as possible, giving the name and position of the staff person involved, and the date, time, place and specific nature of the infraction. Unless the patient has suffered serious injury as a result, we will ensure better care in the future by asking for an explanation rather than demanding retribution.

Family and friends have a legitimate right to be concerned about a patient's care and to question hospital staff about treatment, but should exercise some caution in their zeal to protect him. When families are overwhelmed with anxiety during a medical crisis, they often create many new problems for the patient. Their anxiety can be expressed in many ways: criticism of all medical staff, suspicion regarding all aspects of care, constant demands for attention and service or arguments with the patient and staff about the treatment program.

Analyzing our own behavior is difficult under any circumstance; when a loved one is seriously ill, it may be virtually impossible. If we are highly critical of everything about the patient's care, we ought to talk to a counsellor who can help us deal with our anxiety. We will be of little value to the patient if we cause him to be anxious or if we alienate the hospital staff who are caring for him.

Paying for Hospital Care

Payment for hospital care can be an overwhelming concern, a worry that makes the patient as sick as his condition does.

Hospitals employ social workers or financial counsellors to help with payment problems, insurance claims and financial-aid resources. Those hospitals that received federal Hill-Burton funds for their construction (over half the hospitals in this country) are required by law to provide some free or reduced-cost care to patients who cannot pay for their own care. Since these arrangements vary with each institution, a counsellor should be consulted soon after a patient's admission if he needs financial help. Unfortunately, most hospitals distribute their annual quota of free care soon after the start of the fiscal year, so many who might qualify are turned down. While few patients in this country are denied emergency care because they lack money, many who require long-term rehabilitation are not so lucky.*

Now that we have some hospital orientation and some idea of how to get information, we can begin to help the patient "play his own ball game." To do this, he needs to increase his independence, responsibility and self-esteem so that he feels in control.

PROMOTING PATIENT INDEPENDENCE

A hospital can make a patient feel very dependent, because its routine demands that he eat, sleep, eliminate wastes and perform a variety of other functions on a schedule that has little to do with his needs as an individual. Hospitals could not function if patients were permitted to eat and sleep when they wish; certain tasks must be completed on each shift. Sometimes, however, we can improve the patient's chances for independence if we help staff with their duties.

> Following a stroke which paralyzed her right side, Mrs. Turner had to use her left hand for eating, a laborious, time-consuming process for which she needed much help. Since the nurse's aides had many other patients to help at mealtime, to speed things up they fed her. After her family observed her distress from being fed "like a baby," as she put it, they planned their visits so one of them could be there for each meal. When thus given time and encouragement to feed herself, Mrs. Turner began to feel more independent.

In other instances where hospital routine seems unnecessarily rigid, to the detriment of the patient, we can ask for a variation in schedule to accommodate his needs:

* For a detailed discussion of insurance and medical benefits and ideas for finding financial assistance, see Chapter 7 below.

The doctors ordered Mr. Spencer to sit in a chair twice each day. For convenience, staff had him sit in his chair each morning and evening when they straightened his bed. Mrs. Spencer noticed that he was being unusually subservient when his employees came to visit in the afternoon. She discussed this with him, and he admitted feeling uncomfortable lying in bed while his employees sat or stood about him. She asked the nurses to let him sit in his chair when he planned to have visitors, and they were happy to oblige.

Hospital staff have good reasons for calling some patients by their first name (because they are children or teenagers or long-term, obviously convivial or disoriented patients), but many find this practice excessive and demeaning. If a patient objects to staff using his first name yet is too timid to complain on his own behalf, his family should ask them to address him by his surname.

Often patients are given unnecessary narcotics or sedatives, when fear causes pain or sleeplessness. Since most staff are too busy to sit with all the patients who need reassurance, they resort to administering pills and injections. Usually the patient is not physically harmed by these drugs (unless excessive and unnecessary use leads to addiction), but they temporarily dull his senses and deprive him of opportunities to learn and gain control. The family should spend time with the patient, helping him to settle his fears, and thus reduce his need for these drugs and increase his chances for independence.

Some families are guilty themselves of promoting dependence during hospitalization; they insist that staff give unneeded care when the patient is supposed to do things for himself, or otherwise express their concern through overprotection. Wives or husbands who have played a submissive role during marriage frequently use their spouse's disability as an opportunity to assume leadership. Mothers who have lost their mothering role as the children have left home often use the disability of a family member as a chance to prove their usefulness once more. If nursing staff suggest that we are doing too much for the patient, we would do well to heed their advice.[6]

Learning Opportunities That Enhance Independence

Hospitals generally give patients many chances to learn about their condition and treatment in order to make intelligent decisions about their own care. Family members should encourage the patient to take advantage of these opportunities and participate with him whenever possible.

Nurses and other hospital staff often hold regular classes to instruct patients and their families. For example, diabetics are taught how to manage the disease, check urine- or blood-sugar levels and administer insulin; patients with colostomies are taught how to care for their equipment and regulate their diet.

In addition, social workers or rehabilitation staff conduct self-help groups for patients with similar conditions. During informal sessions, patients and their relatives discuss their concerns and learn how others have coped with the same kinds of problems. These counselling sessions are extremely valuable because the patient comes to see that he has choices and can make his own decisions.

Volunteer visitor services provide another important learning opportunity. Volunteers who have successfully adjusted to their own disabilities visit patients with similar conditions to offer reassurance and encouragement. Reach to Recovery, for example, is a national organization sponsored by the American Cancer Society and composed of women who have had mastectomies. They visit patients after surgery to give woman-to-woman counselling. Less formally organized visitors provide this service to other types of patients. Doctors or nurses arrange for visitor counselling when they feel the patient is not responding to treatment because he thinks his condition is hopeless. Family members can and should ask them to enlist a volunteer if they suspect that the patient needs some encouragement.

> Almost a year after my daughter Lisa's accident, her oral surgeon asked her to visit a young woman who was newly hospitalized with facial injuries similar to hers. During their visits, Lisa answered her questions—such as, "Didn't that hurt?" "How long before these bones healed?" "How did it feel when they took out these screws?"—with the voice of experience. From pictures that Lisa brought along, the young woman could clearly see the progress Lisa had made in the course of a year. Seeing Lisa's results and knowing what to expect from her treatments strengthened her courage to face the months ahead.

Hospital dietitians are a valuable resource for patients on special diets, as well as family members responsible for meal preparation. They help the patient follow his diet by involving him in menu planning and accommodating him as regards food preferences whenever possible. They supply helpful pamphlets about menus and recipes and often suggest inexpensive sources for special foods.

When the patient is receiving treatment that will continue after hospital discharge, family should ask to observe or participate in these procedures if he will need help at home. By closely watching the nurse or therapist, they can learn how to help and when to encourage him to do things for himself.

> Mr. Douglas was eager to take his wife home from the hospital because he knew she would improve faster in familiar surroundings. But he was afraid he would not be able to manage with her bladder catheter. When he mentioned his concern to a nurse, she taught him how to administer the catheter. He practised under her supervision until he was comfortable with his newly acquired skills.

Our closeness to the patient can sometimes hinder our effectiveness as caretakers:

> Despite my own training as a nurse, many aspects of Lisa's care frightened me because my feelings as a mother interfered with my knowledge and judgment as a nurse. Yet I knew I would be responsible for her care when we took her home. Her nurses understood my feelings and gave me many opportunities to help with her care so I could regain my confidence.

Although some hospitals still provide only recreational and inspirational reading materials in their patient libraries, many now maintain collections of medical information for circulation to patients and their families. If this service is not available, doctors or nurses can often supply or recommend helpful publications.

There is nothing magical about the practice of medicine. All of us have the ability to acquire nursing skills and understand disease if we take advantage of learning opportunities. As the patient and his family learn, his capacity to be independent and make decisions about his care increases.

Encouraging Patient Responsibility

Consumer and professional groups have made great strides in promoting patient responsibility, but many patients still refuse to take part in decisions about their care. Usually these people have never bothered to set goals for themselves; instead, they have drifted along, expending little energy or thought towards influencing the outcome of their lives. Encouraging such a patient to take responsibility and set goals for his treatment program is extremely difficult. Nevertheless, family members should still try to get him involved in making decisions about his treatment.

Goal setting plays an important part in planning treatment, so both patient and family ought to understand the steps in this process. The first step involves appraisal by medical staff of what the patient can realistically accomplish within the restrictions of his disability. Professionals admit that they do not always know what to expect or that their assessment and prediction may well prove wrong; but their views, reflecting previous experience, provide a base on which to build.

Professional staff then reaches some agreement with the patient about goals for treatment. When the patient refuses to acknowledge his limitations or feels the professional goals conflict with his own, he will resist their prescribed program. In rare instances, professional staff may set goals according to the needs of the institution rather than the patient. For example, patients are sometimes discharged prematurely, to make space for others; or they are taught skills that help the hospital routine but have little to do with their needs when they eventually go home.

It is important that family agree with the goals set by the patient and staff, in order to wholeheartedly encourage the patient's cooperation. Family attitudes that are too optimistic or pessimistic can sabotage the best treatment program.

For all these reasons, a frank discussion about treatment goals involving staff, patient and family is absolutely essential. It will reveal differences, if they exist, and should help everyone reach a consensus before proceeding to other decisions.

Finally, goals for treatment should be broken down into short-term objectives that will be easy for the patient to accomplish and will help him to reach his final destination. Such short-term objectives are especially important when the patient is severely disabled and faces prolonged treatment. As he accomplishes each intermediate objective—relearning to use a spoon, gaining the strength to sit in a chair, or going through a painful procedure—he gains the confidence to take the next, possibly more difficult, step.

A bedside calendar can be useful in helping someone to tolerate difficult treatments and set time limits for completing objectives. Pointing to the calendar, one can say, "Look, the doctors think those

tubes will come out on Thursday, and then you can drink some liq-
uids," or, "I know you're dreading your next operation because the
first two days after surgery will be painful, but see, by this time next
week the worst will be over and you'll have passed another major
hurdle."

> When Lisa finally realized that she faced several operations and
> months of treatment, we helped her set up a calendar on which
> she recorded anticipated dates for the completion of her objec-
> tives. At each milestone—for example, whenever she relearned a
> skill, received a new cast or recovered from another operation—
> we celebrated by taking her photograph. By documenting her
> progress in this fashion, we helped her appreciate her tremendous
> accomplishments. This evidence made her want to work harder.

The use of a calendar is almost always appropriate for long-term
patients, although a camera might offend some people. Both are valuable tools because they focus the patient's attention on short-term,
easily reachable objectives. If he concentrates on these objectives he
is less apt to become depressed than if he thinks only about the long
path to recovery.

When the patient takes part in setting realistic long- and short-
term goals and treatment objectives, he makes a commitment to
himself and others involved in his care, a commitment that increases his sense of responsibility and gives his life a purpose.

Restoring Self-confidence

Disability can destroy an individual's self-confidence; he tends to
feel worthless, isolated, angry, guilty and afraid. Until he can overcome these feelings, they will threaten his recovery and adjustment
to disability. Fortunately, we can do a great deal during hospitalization to help him cope with these feelings and regain self-confidence.

Many people dislike talking about their feelings under any circumstances, usually because they think they will appear weak.
When disability strikes, even those who are generally more open
have difficulty discussing their feelings, because those feelings can
be so ugly and discomforting.

We can help even those patients who think they are strong and
emotionally self-sufficient by listening carefully and non-judgmen-
tally to what they say. When a patient expresses deep-seated feelings, we can say, for example, "It's alright for you to feel angry," "I
understand why you're afraid," or, "Tell me why you're feeling

guilty." If he is encouraged to talk openly about his feelings, he will be able to deal with them constructively; if they remain buried, they will fester and cripple him emotionally.

Hospital staff often suggest professional counselling when a patient's emotional problems are hampering his recovery. But since staff are not apt to be familiar with the patient's usual behavior, they may not recognize symptoms of distress that are obvious to his family. If we think he needs help in coping with his feelings, we can ask the doctor to refer him to someone for counselling. Most hospitals have a variety of staff personnel who are trained to help patients, including psychologists, social workers and clergy. Usually the patient can choose the type of counsellor he prefers.

A distressed patient often will not need professional help, however, if he can find a way to get things off his chest. A diary can be especially useful in this regard, because it helps the patient to bring feelings to a conscious level where they can be dealt with.

> Shortly after Lisa's accident, friends gave her a notebook for recording her daily progress. The empty pages soon became a basket into which Lisa dumped the ugly feelings she couldn't express to anyone else. As she recorded her thoughts and examined them, she found they were not so terrible, after all.

In addition to needing help in coping with these feelings, patients need to be reminded of their personal value. Such reminders will give self-confidence a tremendous boost.

> Mrs. Billings was grateful for her family's frequent visits and somewhat relieved to learn they could manage at home without her. But seeing how easily her husband and children had taken over her mothering duties, she soon felt useless and depressed. When her family discovered the cause of her depression, they decided to put her to work. Her husband asked for help with the checkbook and bill payments; her daughter sought advice about household routine; and her son brought his homework to the hospital so she could help him. Mrs. Billings was delighted with their demands for help, because she realized she was important to her family even when confined to a hospital bed.

When the patient's condition permits, simple recreational activities help to pass the time, remind him of remaining abilities and make him feel good about himself. Books, puzzles, games, or arts and crafts are all useful here. Projects can be designed to fit individual needs. For example, a grandmother might enjoy arranging a long-neglected family album, in part because the pictures remind her of her status in the family.

> Mr. Lee, a professional guitarist, shared a hospital room with another young man, who was eager to learn to play the guitar. Since both men expected long confinement, they received permission to have two guitars brought to the hospital. Soon Mr. Lee's pupil was playing simple tunes; their practice sessions quickly attracted an appreciative audience of ambulatory patients.

When people become disabled they often worry about their sex lives, fearing failure and rejection. At the very time when they most need assurances of love, demonstrations of intimacy are usually prohibited by hospital routine and regulations. Although some rehabilitation centers now have "privacy rooms," most acute-care institutions do not permit conjugal visits, because they lack the space and scheduling flexibility for such activities. Occasionally, regulations are relaxed so that the patient can have uninterrupted privacy with his visitor. If a patient faces a long hospitalization and appears to need some sexual gratification, the staff should be asked to provide some privacy, if at all possible.

> After Mr. Taylor's leg was amputated, he most feared that his wife would find his disfigurement sexually repulsive. Having been married to him for thirty-nine years, she sensed his concern, and, casting aside her embarrassment, spoke to his nurse. With some minor adjustments in routine and cautions about his condition, the nurse arranged for the couple to be alone while his roommate was out for a treatment. The hospital commandment, "No visitor shall sit on a patient's bed," was disobeyed in the extreme, but Mr. Taylor's spirits were rapidly revived.

> After Mrs. Lewis was badly disfigured in an accident, understanding nurses regularly arranged for her husband to have time alone with her. They recognized that his cuddles and caresses would do more to ensure her recovery than all the treatment they could provide.

When it is impossible for a patient's sexual needs to be gratified in the hospital, he should at least receive assurances of love. He needs to know that he is still the most valuable person in his partner's life.

People who lose their ability to communicate, temporarily or permanently, feel isolated and inferior because they can no longer participate in conversations or express their needs. Hospital staff are usually eager to help such patients; they supply tools for other forms of communication and explain to family how they can help the patient. Simple aids—paper and pencil, a "magic slate," charts or cards—will help, depending upon his needs.

> Mr. Ferguson could neither speak nor write for a time after his surgery, so his grandchildren constructed large charts. In each space they printed a sentence, such as "I'm hungry," "I'm thirsty," or "How's my garden doing?" One morning when a nurse announced that it was time for his bath, he grabbed a chart and emphatically-pointed to one of its phrases. The nurse laughed as she read, "I'd rather be fishing." With his ability to communicate partially restored, he had regained his sense of humor.

An individual who loses his ability to communicate usually still retains all the qualities of his personality; but he often appears to be less than he was because he cannot share those qualities with us. When we are familiar with a person and can tap such inner resources as humor, kindness and intelligence, we give his self-confidence a tremendous lift.

Many hospitals provide translation services for patients who only speak a foreign language. If necessary, family members can devise simple cards or charts with pictures or bilingual phrases for the patient to use in their absence.

There is a tendency to ignore individuals with communication problems. Whenever possible, we should include the patient in conversations, resorting to gestures or pad and pencil if need be. When the patient appears to be in a coma, we ought to behave as though he can hear and understand what we say. Disoriented patients demand our utmost patience; we can only hope that our repeated reassurances will relieve their distress and help to improve their condition in time.

Like the rest of us, patients feel better when they are comfortable about their appearance and in pleasant surroundings. Our small efforts in this regard will greatly improve a patient's morale. To this end, we can offer to help with shaving or hair care, encourage a woman patient to use cosmetics or supply her with feminine gowns or robes to wear. For a long-term patient with a cast or other special equipment, we can modify the clothing temporarily by splitting seams and attaching ties or other fasteners. A patient will often feel better if he can wear his own clothing, but we must be willing to do his laundry ourselves when he chooses to wear non-regulation attire; the hospital will not do it.

Finally, small personal additions to a hospital room help restore the patient's self-confidence, because they enable him to carve out a personal space of his own. Flowers, plants, family photographs, drawings from young children, posters, stuffed animals or an attractive display of greeting cards all brighten the room and remind him that he is a valuable person to his family and friends.

TIPS FOR HOSPITAL VISITORS

Many people unthinkingly rush to visit a friend or relative who is hospitalized. Visitors are potentially beneficial, but they frequently cause problems. Sometimes they congregate in large groups, obstructing staff routine, interfering with treatment and disturbing the comfort and privacy of other patients. They may use their visits to socialize with other friends and relatives, showing little concern for the patient.

Hospital visits require careful planning. First, we must consider our relationship to the patient and his condition. For example, only immediate family or very close friends should be with the patient when he is acutely ill. Immediate family should suggest to friends or other relatives when they may visit, and, if the patient is bothered by unwanted visitors, should ask for visiting restrictions.

Those who are not immediate family would best direct their concern for the critically ill patient towards helping his family. There will be plenty of time during convalescence when the patient will need company. In the meantime, they can offer to perform tasks for the immediate family or keep them company while they are at the hospital but cannot be with the patient. When families must spend long hours in waiting rooms, they are invariably grateful for the diversion and comfort of sympathetic friends.

Many hospitals have lenient visiting hours lasting from midmorning to early evening, but, since a patient may require many treatments during a day, it is a good idea to ask the nursing staff when the patient is likely to be available for visitors. No matter how carefully we plan our visits, there will be times when our presence in the room interferes with the patient's care or infringes on the privacy of other patients in the room. Even when not asked, we should graciously leave the room. Anyone who has been a patient and tried to use a bedpan while visitors converse on the other side of a curtain will heartily endorse this advice.

Finally, we ought to consider our hospital visits as opportunities for helping the patient. Certainly there are times when he needs only our engaging conversation and congenial company, but often we can perform tasks that will enhance the value of our visit. For example, we can run errands, read aloud, help with correspondence or play games to help him pass the time. If the staff is agreeable, we can take him on walks in the hall or visits to the lounge, hospital chapel or gift shop. When we help the patient with his special needs, we break the pattern of the traditional hospital visit by showing him that he is an important individual rather than just another "hospital patient."

Incidentally, hospitals often provide a number of services for the comfort and convenience of visitors: waiting rooms, often staffed by volunteers, for family use when the patient is in surgery or on a critical-care unit; gift shops, cafeterias and chapel facilities; and information centers, with, for example, listings of inexpensive motels and rooming houses and bulletin boards where visitors can arrange for carpooling.

PLANNING FOR DISCHARGE

Discharge planning is an important hospital function, second only to providing care during hospitalization. Ideally, it should start when the patient is admitted to the hospital; treatment goals, after all, must be directed towards eventual discharge. Sometimes few plans are needed; at the time of discharge the patient is given simple instructions about medication, diet and exercise, told when to return to his doctor and carefully ushered to the exit. For patients with severe disability, however, the planning process is complex.

Many things must be considered in deciding when a patient is ready for discharge and where he will go afterwards. These include his condition and further treatment needs; his ability to return home and the family's ability to care for him, if necessary; and the availability of community resources to meet his needs. The patient and his family must be involved in this planning from the outset, because they have so much at stake in these decisions.

Specialized nursing staff within the hospital are responsible for coordinating discharge planning. Although titles vary depending on the institution—"discharge planning nurse," "liaison nurse," "continuing care nurse" or "utilization review coordinator"—these workers assess the patient's condition and family circumstances and make necessary arrangements for care after discharge. They work closely with hospital social workers to make referrals, secure financial assistance and locate community services.

Early discharge is now encouraged because of rising hospital costs, and, in some areas, bed shortages. For the most part, patients benefit from this practice, since it promotes self-reliance. For those who are able to live at home but continue to need treatment, public health nursing departments, private home health-care agencies and metropolitan hospitals provide care in the form of visiting nurses, therapists and other professionals; and almost all hospitals maintain out-patient services for those who need such periodic treatments as physical therapy, chemotherapy or renal (kidney) dialysis.

Recently the New York University Medical Center opened an innovative cooperative-care unit to prepare patients and their families for early discharge. In this unit, an appropriate family member or close friend shares the patient's room for a few days prior to discharge to learn how to care for the patient at home. Irvin G. Wilmot, executive vice-president of the center, says, "We're altering the traditional patterns of hospital care. . . . In the past we've said, 'Go to the hospital, get in bed. We'll take care of you.' This kind of service furthers dependency. We're trying to move the patient towards an independent state earlier."[7] Although few of us have access to this sort of transition facility, we can prepare ourselves to assume our relative's care by being alert and inquisitive during his hospital stay.

Hospital discharge comes as a welcome relief to most patients, but it can seem threatening to a long-term patient who has become dependent on staff for many services. Such a patient fears the loss of established routine and the problems he will face at home. However, if we who are close to him have done a good job during his hospitalization, he will anticipate discharge with confidence, knowing that it represents another milestone in his recovery.

CHAPTER 3

Rehabilitation Alternatives

IN ONE SENSE, REHABILITATION BEGINS the minute an individual discovers he is disabled. But the real work of rehabilitation starts after the acute phase of illness or injury has passed—after medication has been properly adjusted, bones and incisions healed and intensive medical treatment completed.

At this point some people leave the hospital, returning home for a brief period of convalescence, after which they will resume normal activity. Some will not be so lucky, being severely disabled; they will need rehabilitation. Since such a patient should receive treatment in a setting that encourages maximum independence, his family and friends ought to be familiar with the rehabilitation process and the types of facilities that offer rehabilitation.

The word "rehabilitation" has many meanings. Since this book considers a wide spectrum of disabling conditions, a definition that is appropriate for any kind of disability is necessary. For our general purposes, then, rehabilitation is a process by which a newly disabled person learns to perform at his highest possible level of activity. This is a broad definition, but one that stresses an outlook essential to successful rehabilitation. Since it does not mention the patient's former, healthy condition, it gives little emphasis on what he has lost. It implies that a person with disability can use his remaining abilities to achieve something more satisfying than he had previously. Rather than looking backwards to how good things were before the patient became disabled, it looks forwards, emphasizing his potential for personal growth.

It should be noted that rehabilitation often requires more than helping the patient adapt to his disability. Conditions in his environment and the attitudes of his associates must also be changed so they do not handicap him. For example, many disabled people are employable but cannot work because they lack transportation or no one will hire them. Insofar as possible then, rehabilitation should change the environment, removing architectural and transportation barriers and creating opportunities for employment and recreation. These efforts are often as important as the patient's treatment.

PSYCHOLOGICAL ASPECTS OF REHABILITATION

Clearly, rehabilitation must mean more than physical restoration. Most rehabilitation workers agree with psychologist Beatrice A. Wright that changing attitudes—of both the patient and those around him—is an important part of rehabilitation.[1] According to Dr. Wright, the patient may need to change his attitudes about what is valuable in his life. He must eventually realize that he can learn new skills that will become as valuable, or more valuable, to him than those he has lost. For example, if he can no longer walk, he must broaden his horizons and develop new abilities that will become as important to him as walking.

Dr. Wright further maintains that the patient may have to lessen the value he places on his body and its abilities, and concentrate instead on his emotional and intellectual qualities. He should remember that although we hold athletes in high esteem, we save our greatest praise for the person who is thoughtful, kind and generous. A disabled body can be retrained to perform old skills or it can learn new ones, but often the greatest potential for growth exists in the mind.

Comparisons between disabled and healthy bodies are unavoidable, but lose significance when we consider the enormous range in appearance and ability among people with normal bodies. Rehabilitation acknowledges differences, but helps the individual to recognize and develop his own abilities without comparing himself to others.

Dr. Wright says that attitudes towards disability tend to "spread," so that a disabled person automatically thinks of himself, and is viewed by others, as being incapable of doing things that in fact have nothing to do with his particular limitations. For example, we might assume that a severely disabled person could not be a good manager simply because he has physical limitations; in fact, he may have excellent managerial capabilities. Rehabilitation can lessen the overall effect of disability on a person's life by confining the influence of the disability to as few activities as possible and emphasizing what the individual *can* do.

The Family's Role

We have seen that family, friends and professional staff can greatly influence how a patient thinks about himself and his disability. According to occupational therapist Hilda P. Versluys, the family becomes especially important as the patient prepares for rehabilitation.

> The role of the family in rehabilitation is crucial. The family's response to the injured or ill person may determine the patient's motivation to tolerate painful procedures and long-term treatment, to face irrevocable losses, and to accept major lifestyle changes.... Excellent treatment programs may never realize their potential due to the collapse of a concerned but overwhelmed family.[2]

Since families are so important in the rehabilitation process, we ought to understand why some families rise to the challenge while others disintegrate when faced with disability. Versluys suggests some answers: Some families seem to handle any sort of crisis well, because their members share affection and communicate freely with one another. By being flexible and willing to change or delay individual goals, family members are able to take on new responsibilities and work towards goals that are important for the whole family. They rearrange schedules so each person has time to "do his own thing." They bolster the patient's confidence by encouraging him to participate in family decisions and jobs. They hold a positive but realistic view of the future. They recognize their own limitations, and ask for help when necessary.

In other families, any crisis can cause new problems for everyone concerned. There is little sharing, support, communication or cooperation; members seem unable to change their goals or take on new responsibilities. They are so overwhelmed by stress and conflict that they resort to damaging behavior despite their best intentions. They may be overprotective, encouraging the patient's dependency in order to increase their own sense of usefulness. They may express their unacknowledged resentment about the patient's condition by being angry at him or rejecting him. They often deny his importance as an individual or family member. They tend to view his condition unrealistically, rejecting his diagnosis and its implications while searching for an instant cure, or instead adopting a pessimistic attitude about chances for recovery. They often place excessive demands upon one another, but refuse to accept responsibility themselves. Sometimes, members leave the family.

Relationships within families are seldom all bad or all good. When we examine our own families, we're likely to find good as well as bad qualities. Even if a family cooperates and communicates well, the problems of disability can cause stresses that members are poorly equipped to handle alone. For this reason, family counselling can be an important part of the patient's rehabilitation.

PLANNING FOR REHABILITATION

Decisions about where the patient will go for rehabilitation treatment largely depend upon the family's ability and willingness to help the patient. There are other factors to consider as well. Those who are planning for rehabilitation—the professional team as well as the patient and family—need to ask themselves these questions:

- What are the eventual goals of rehabilitation? Does everyone agree that they are possible to achieve?
- What forms of treatment are required to reach these goals?
- Is the family emotionally and physically able to provide these services, or can treatment only be supplied by an institution?
- Are resources available in the community to help the family care for the patient?
- Are other appropriate care facilities available if the family cannot assume the patient's care?

- What are the family's financial circumstances? Do
  they limit the family's choices?

Lack of money undoubtedly limits choices, but here it deserves to be the last consideration, because it has nothing to do with deciding what is best for the patient. Once agreement is reached about rehabilitation needs, then ways to pay for the care can be investigated.

TYPES OF FACILITIES

A doctor is likely to recommend treatment in a rehabilitation facility if the patient is severely disabled and requires many services. The American Hospital Association classifies these facilities into four types: completely independent rehabilitation hospitals; self-contained rehabilitation hospitals within large medical centers; defined rehabilitation units within hospitals; and hospitals that provide rehabilitation services but have no formalized units.[3]

The purpose of a rehabilitation facility, naturally, determines its services and staff; programs for treating patients with spinal cord injuries are quite different from those that help deaf people. In general, most facilities employ a team of physiatrists, therapists, psychologists, social workers, nurses and other professionally trained personnel.

Physiatrists are doctors who have specialized in physical medicine and rehabilitation; they usually direct the treatment program.

Physical therapists are responsible for physical restoration. Employing a variety of equipment, they use massage and regulated exercise to improve coordination and balance, reeducate muscles, restore joint motion and increase the patient's tolerance for activity.

Occupational therapists help the patient to develop skills associated with daily living, such as dressing, eating and grooming. After carefully assessing the patient's needs, they design techniques and use adaptive equipment to enhance his abilities. Facilities often include a model bathroom and kitchen in which patients can practice daily living skills. In addition, these therapists work with families and employers to suggest modifications in the patient's home and work environment.

Psychologists and social workers are primarily concerned with the emotional aspects of rehabilitation. Through individual and group counselling, they help patients and their families to develop healthy attitudes, adjust to changes in lifestyle and prepare for hospital discharge. Depending on the scope of the center, they may also furnish vocational counselling, testing and placement services. Many facilities also have staff chaplains trained to assist with patient and family counselling.

Other members of the professional team include, but are not limited to, rehabilitation nurses, brace and limb specialists, speech and recreation therapists, dietitians and discharge-planning nurses.

Evaluating a Facility

A doctor's choice of facility for a patient will depend upon his own experiences, the needs of the patient and the location of suitable services. Although often a patient can receive the care he needs from a local institution, at other times transfer to a center specializing in a particular condition is desirable. If we question the doctor's recommendation or want to explore other possibilities, the guidelines below will help to evaluate a facility.[4]

In a highly qualified rehabilitation facility, treatment is directed towards returning the patient to his family or community rather than providing custodial care. Such a facility will have a comprehensive program of services that meets all the patient's needs, provided by a qualified staff of consultants or full-time specialists. The staff will encourage family education and cooperation, and hold regular team conferences to involve the patient and family in treatment decisions. They will be supportive, sensitive and honest. Provisions for treatment will include referral and follow-up after discharge.

Beyond being clean and attractive, a rehabilitation facility ought to be designed so that patients have privacy, but are not isolated from life on the unit. Having separate, easily accessible space for treatment and for social activity is essential. A friendly, homelike environment where patients can participate in meal preparation and group dining is desirable. And there should be opportunity for socializing both on and off the unit.

Rehabilitation centers with good programs, well-qualified staff and adequate facilities are accredited by the Joint Commission on Accreditation of Hospitals and the Commission on Accreditation of Rehabilitation Facilities (CARF). Any facility meeting the standards of these two groups probably provides high-quality care, although its services may not be appropriate for a particular disability.*

* For help in locating a suitable treatment facility, contact a nearby university medical center, or write to CARF at 2500 N. Pantano Road, Tucson AZ 85715.

Family Involvement on the Rehabilitation Unit

Treatment in a formal rehabilitation setting should be the first choice for a severely disabled patient; sometimes it is the only appropriate option. Other alternatives can be considered in some cases, but only after the patient has been thoroughly evaluated by a competent rehabilitation team. The advantages of excellent services provided in a distant facility must often be weighed against the patient's need for family support.[5] Many patients are sufficiently independent, strong and determined to manage well without close family contact; others progress far more rapidly when near their families, even if they thereby have fewer and less adequate professional services.

Families tend to view the time the patient spends in a rehabilitation facility as a honeymoon—a period when the initial crisis has passed, but they are not yet responsible for his care.[6] The patient, however, continues to need his family's support as much as ever. Through frequent visits, large doses of praise and assurances of love, they can persist in building his self-confidence. Whenever possible, they should participate in his treatments in order to learn how to help and when to encourage independence. And finally, family members should work closely with his rehabilitation staff to plan for discharge.

Despite careful preparation, discharge from a rehabilitation unit can be devastating. For the patient, discharge means the medical profession has done everything it can for him—and he is apt to be disappointed with the results. He fears his family will be unable to care for him properly, and that his dependence will make him low man on the family totem pole. Conversely, family members may question their ability to care for him. To test circumstances in the home, patients should be encouraged to take weekend passes. Rehabilitation staff can then help to resolve difficulties before the patient is permanently discharged.

REHABILITATION TREATMENT AT HOME

Families can provide excellent rehabilitative care at home—sometimes even when the patient is severely disabled—if they have suitable advice and help. Home care may require vast amounts of planning and effort, but the compensations are often great. In their book, *The Rehabilitation Environment*, psychologists Carroll Brodsky and Robert Platt explain,

The major distinction between family and institutional care is that the family establishes its rehabilitation program for one purpose only—to rehabilitate an individual who is very important to them. On the other hand, the hospital rehabilitation unit is established to meet a spectrum of needs including those of institutions, community, teachers, patients and staff. . . . It is difficult to design an institution that provides an optimal social and psychological environment and virtually impossible to design one that provides the kind of love, care, interest and participation that is found in the family.[7]

Advantages and Disadvantages of Home Care

In an emotionally healthy family, the patient benefits from being in familiar surroundings. He has closer contact with his family and friends, a flexible schedule and more personalized attention. His sense of well-being is greatly enhanced by continuous love and support and encouragement to participate in family activities.

Conversely, the patient suffers at home in a family where his care causes disruptive changes and stress. He will feel helpless if the arrangement of his home limits his movement, and isolated if his family limits his social contacts because they are embarrassed by his condition. Finally, his rehabilitation may be seriously threatened if the family fails to carry out treatment orders because they lack adequate instruction or supervision.

Home care can be far less expensive than institutional treatment, but the actual costs to the family will depend upon the patient's eligibility for insurance and other benefits. He may be entitled to medical benefits only when hospitalized. On the other hand, his coverage may include expenses for out-patient treatment; visiting professional services, equipment and supplies; and medical transportation. If he lacks coverage for home care expenses, or a family member must quit work to care for him, home care may cost the family more than institutional care.

Preparations for Home Care

It is impossible to make an intelligent decision about whether to undertake home care without knowing what that task involves. Good intentions are not enough. Besides the cost, we need to know how to prepare ourselves and the home for the patient, and where to go for help. We need to have a clear understanding of the treatment program and what that will entail in terms of time, skills and stamina. Planning for home care must outline clearly what our responsibilities will be.

Before any plans are made, a rehabilitation team must assess the patient's condition in order to determine his needs and decide if the family is capable of providing adequate care. Beyond that, the patient should have a good relationship with the family members who will be caring for him, and must be willing to participate in his treatment. If he has healthy attitudes about his disability and a desire for independence, he is likely to be an ideal candidate for home treatment.

Home nursing skills can easily be learned from a public-health or visiting nurse, who can demonstrate how to perform procedures, set up a daily treatment routine and suggest ways for the patient to help with his care. In addition, specialized books about home nursing techniques can be excellent guides.

In an institutional setting, the patient's progress is closely monitored by professional staff. At home, unless other arrangements are made, we are responsible for observing and reporting important changes. This task is not so difficult, because we have only one patient and can easily learn what to observe. Before our relative comes home, we should ask his doctor about medication and treatment so we understand their purpose and can recognize unfavorable symptoms. We should also find out exactly how to reach the doctor—where and when to call—in case we have problems. Most doctors take time to discuss these matters, because they know that our confidence in them will improve the patient's care.

Patients on a rigorous schedule of treatment often need more care than their family can provide. Doctors, hospital social workers and discharge-planning nurses or public health nurses can help locate outside help when necessary.* If, on the other hand, the patient needs frequent treatments at his doctor's office or a hospital, we will have to arrange for transportation, be it by ambulance, taxi or other service or by a relative, friend or neighbor.

Medicines and medical supplies are other things to consider in planning for home care. Although these items are expensive, ways can be found to reduce their cost. For example, doctors can often prescribe drugs by generic rather than brand name, or suggest pharmacies that charge reasonable prices for drugs and other supplies; otherwise it is worthwhile to do some comparative shopping. Community agencies sometimes provide sickroom supplies and medica-

* See Chapter 5 for more information about these resources.

tion free or at greatly reduced cost to patients with particular conditions. For instance, some local chapters of the American Cancer Society dispense surgical dressings and medications to cancer patients. Public health nurses are a good source for this kind of information.

We should organize the home so that the patient will feel safe and comfortable and we can care for him with a minimum of effort. Public health nurses and occupational therapists can help with these arrangements or suggest necessary home modifications. If the patient is confined to bed most of the time, he should have a room that is conveniently located yet private—ideally, near a bathroom for him or anyone who has to tote a bedpan and bathwater. Although privacy is important, some patients who are confined to bed want to be in the middle of family activity; in that case, a living room or dining room could be converted into a temporary bedroom. In any event, the room selected ought to be cheerful, well lighted and ventilated, with a view to the outside.[8]

Hospital-discharge-planning nurses and public health nurses can help locate specialized equipment, including a hospital bed for the patient's comfort and our convenience in giving care; flotation mattress to prevent bedsores; an over-the-bed table for eating and other activities; hydraulic lift for transferring the patient from bed to chair; wheelchair, walker or crutches. In addition to local businesses that rent sickroom equipment, nursing organizations, fire departments and service groups often maintain supplies of equipment for free loan.

Sometimes, of course, it is possible to improvise with the furnishings on hand. While making sure to remove all unnecessary clutter from the patient's room, we may want to add some things: a bedside table for storing personal and frequently used items; a bell or other device to call for help; a bedside commode; perhaps a reading light, telephone, radio and television. Our goal is to give the patient every possible opportunity for independence. When his movement is restricted, little things count. Every time he can reach for a water glass, change a television channel or adjust the lighting in the room, he gains a sense of mastery over his environment. But each time he has to call for help because something is out of reach, he feels dependent and worthless.

Preparations for home rehabilitation care will be different for each person, but they are always necessary. During the planning process, we must evaluate our abilities and resources to decide if we are equipped to handle the job. We may decide to accept the challenge despite great emotional, physical and financial sacrifice. Or we may have no choice but to accept it. Whatever our reasons, we will reduce our work and worry considerably if we prepare the patient, our home and ourselves beforehand.*

REHABILITATION AT A NURSING HOME

Nursing homes are an alternative for rehabilitation care when the patient lacks a family or his family cannot care for him. Unfortunately, many people think of nursing homes as warehouses where old people are left to die. If the patient who is admitted to a nursing home happens to share this view, he will feel hopeless and abandoned. We must do everything we can to help him feel otherwise.

Choosing a nursing home for a loved one is a difficult task, as anyone who has been through that experience knows. The choice is complicated by the variety in nursing homes, services they offer and quality of care. The goals of the patient ought to be the foremost consideration in selecting a nursing home. If he hopes to return home someday, and these hopes are realistic, we need to find a facility that offers rehabilitation treatment.

Nursing homes are state licensed to provide specific kinds of care. Some are licensed for *skilled care*—that is, medical and rehabilitative treatment by licensed professionals. Others are authorized to give a variety of levels of *custodial care,* such as bathing, feeding, dressing or other assistance. The majority of nursing-home residents receive only custodial care.

Most nursing homes offer some form of physical and occupational therapy, but we cannot assume that therapy services are adequate just because they are offered. Often these services are designed to maintain residents at their present level of function rather than aggressively promote rehabilitation for eventual discharge. However, some homes provide programs appropriate for patients who need a very long treatment period.

Evaluating a Nursing Home

A doctor's recommendation can be helpful in choosing a nursing home, but many physicians have little contact with these institutions. We should do some investigating on our own.

* Many of the ideas in Chapter 4 below, which suggest ways to help the patient during convalescence, apply to the rehabilitation period, especially when the patient is at home. Also applicable is Chapter 6, which looks at methods for coping with stress when caring for a disabled person.

Judging by the number of nursing-home consumer advocate groups in this country, there are many problems associated with nursing homes. Sadly, the ones that give excellent care are in the minority. As with hospitals, there is evidence that non-profit facilities (such as those of the Seventh-Day Adventists) offer better care. Since they have no need to show a profit to stockholders, they provide far superior service for the reimbursement they receive from Medicare and Medicaid (the primary sources of income for nursing homes).[9] The National Citizens' Coalition for Nursing Home Reform* publishes useful guidelines for nursing-home evaluation; nursing-home ombudsman programs in many states also furnish helpful advice.[10] In general, these groups suggest that families examine inspection reports and licenses and personally visit the nursing home to talk with staff and residents and their families.

Nursing homes certified to receive reimbursement from Medicare and Medicaid are inspected regularly; these inspection reports are available for public review. Reports for Medicare-approved facilities are stored at Social Security Administration regional offices; those for Medicaid-approved nursing homes are available upon request from state health departments. These reports may suggest problems to look for when making a personal inspection. Most guidelines advise that an evaluation include the following:

- a review of fire- and health-inspection reports and licensing documents
- an inspection of all parts of the facility, including the kitchen, laundry, bathrooms and treatment and activity areas, with particular attention to cleanliness and fire-prevention and other safety features
- a conference with staff concerning their professional qualifications, treatment services, staffing patterns on each shift and methods for involving residents and their families in treatment decisions
- a review of policies and procedures regarding medical emergencies, admission of patients, segregation of residents with different needs, and room assignments
- a review of regulations for resident conduct, visiting and pass privileges, smoking, drinking and telephone calls

* 1424 16th Street, N.W., Suite 204, Washington, D.C. 20036.

- observations regarding the general appearance of
  the facility, appearance and activities of residents,
  and interaction between staff and residents
- conversations with residents and their families regarding staff attitudes, food service and activity
  programs

Many people are appalled by the suggestion that they visit a
nursing home to conduct an on-the-spot investigation of the facility.
They fear that their questions about safety, services or treatment
procedures constitute an attack on the nursing home. Yet often
these same people would not entrust the safety of a family member
to a used car under consideration for purchase until they had kicked
the tires, tested the brakes, had a friendly mechanic give the car a
careful inspection and consulted its former owners about performance and operational problems. When we entrust a relative to a
nursing home, we are purchasing a service; we have every right to
question the quality of that service. Staff of a nursing home that
offers good care will be proud to show its facilities and inspection
documents, and delighted to have residents interviewed.

At the very start, then, we can feel reassured about a nursing
home if its staff is cooperative in our evaluation of the facility. Satis-
fied testimony from residents and their families is an excellent indication that the staff is kind and the level of custodial care good. As
regards judgments about treatment programs, however, we will
have to rely on professionals who have had experience with these
services.

Nursing homes are not as expensive as hospitals, but their fee
schedules and acceptable methods of payment should be checked
before a disabled relative is admitted to a facility. Almost always,
extra charges are made for medicine, medical supplies and equipment, and special services. Insurance policies frequently pay benefits only for *skilled* care in a *skilled* nursing home for a *specified
time* immediately following hospitalization. Most insurance policies, including "nursing-home insurance" policies, do not pay for
custodial care. Medicare covers some medically prescribed skilled-
care costs, and most Medicare supplement insurance policies pay
additional sums. But the full cost of care is never covered by Medicare. Only people eligible for Medicaid under state guidelines (because they have no money for their own medical care) receive
nursing-home coverage for *both* skilled and custodial care.

If we have no alternative but to send a relative to an inadequate
nursing home, we should monitor his care closely and compensate

for shortcomings through frequent visits. Even when nursing-home conditions are ideal, however, we ought to visit regularly and do everything possible to give him support. Insofar as regulations permit, we can bring him personal mementos from home, encourage self-care and participation in activities with other residents, help maintain outside interests and take him on passes for short excursions or weekend visits. And if discharge is a realistic possibility, we should help him plan for that eventuality.

FURTHER REHABILITATION ALTERNATIVES

Institutional care is not the only choice when a patient is without family and lives alone—if his treatment needs are minimal and suitable support services are available. Many people thrive when they can maintain some degree of independence. One study has found that patients with chronic but moderate disabilities recover more quickly at home, even when living alone, than in nursing homes.[11]

The availability of support services depends upon the community in which a person lives and his reservoir of family contacts, friends and neighbors. In many communities, agencies supply meals, health care, chore and homemaking assistance, and transportation for the homebound disabled and elderly. Sometimes, however, the patient may have a close friend who can move in with him to provide temporary help, or a group of neighbors willing to join forces to provide necessary services.

Medicare, Medicaid and some private insurance companies reimburse the costs of *skilled* home health-care services; they do not pay for the unskilled but highly valuable services that help many people to remain at home alone. It is still cheaper in some states for those who cannot afford medical care to obtain nursing-home care under Medicaid than to receive inexpensive, unskilled support services at home. Some states and insurance companies are trying to change this situation, but progress is slow. In rare instances, it is possible to negotiate with an insurance company or a government agency for payment of unskilled support services when the only alternative is admission into a nursing home.

Foster homes and halfway houses are other possibilities for people with treatment needs who cannot live alone because they require some supervision and assistance. Public health nurses and social workers are familiar with local services of this nature. Personal attendants are another option for people who can afford to hire help. Other types of living arrangements are sometimes available, but most can be considered only after rehabilitation treatment has been completed.*

Rehabilitation has a different meaning for each patient with a disability. Whatever his condition, however, our goal should be to help him find good treatment in an environment that will best encourage his independence.

* See Chapter 6 below for more information about attendant care and independent living facilities.

CHAPTER 4

Putting Convalescent Time to Work

CONVALESCENCE IS BORING. Whatever excitement there was to hospitalization has passed, and the friends who flocked to the bedside are now seeking other diversions. Despite all the anticipation of homecoming, actual reunion with the family resurrects petty annoyances. Now that treatment is almost complete—which does not necessarily mean that *recovery* is complete—the patient thinks, "This is it! This is how I'm going to be for the rest of my life!" He feels useless because time hangs heavy on his hands, and he becomes depressed. Now, more than any other time since the onset of disability, we can help our relative take charge of his life—by putting his convalescent time to work.

THE IMPACT OF DISABILITY

The impact of disability is like that of a rock thrown into a quiet pond. The water is roiled at the point of impact, greatly distorting reflections, and shock waves travel out in concentric circles of decreasing intensity until they reach the shore. When disability strikes, the images a person has of himself and his relationships with those very close to him are greatly disturbed. The shock waves of his disability extend out to affect his dealings with other relatives, friends, casual acquaintances and even strangers. The convalescent period is an ideal time to begin mending the disturbances in each of these circles of relationships.

The view we have of ourselves is largely the reflection of others' behavior towards us; we see ourselves in others' eyes, as the saying goes. When people behave as though they think we are intelligent and good-looking, we feel confident about our appearance and actions. On the other hand, people can easily destroy our self-confidence when they act as though we are ugly or immature. Similarly, disabled people are strongly influenced by the treatment they receive from those around them. The more they value a person, the stronger that influence will be. When the relationship is an intimate one, a sexual one, their partner's reaction towards them and their disability is critical to self-esteem. Unfortunately, sexual relationships are often seriously disturbed, if not destroyed, by disability.

SEX AND THE DISABLED

Today, when sexual pleasure is usually associated with young and beautiful bodies—or at least healthy ones—having fully functional sexual organs, most of us prefer to think of disabled or aged people as sexless. We become uncomfortable imagining that someone who is deformed, aged or retarded is interested in—or, worse yet, occupied with—sex. So, if we ignore the subject of sex, people who are disabled will not think about it. Right?

Wrong. Numerous studies of severely disabled people have shown that sex is an overwhelming concern to them. Some patients are more upset by the loss of their sexual relationships than by their disability.[1] Others say they would prefer retaining their normal sex function to being able to walk again, if given a choice.[2] While research on female sexuality is relatively new, ample evidence shows that disabled women are just as worried about sex as disabled men.[3]

Causes of Sexual Problems

The causes of sexual problems are almost as numerous as the people who suffer from them. Physical limitation, pain and loss of sensation can affect sexual desire or hamper performance. And seemingly minor medical conditions and certain drugs can also be at fault. Mental attitudes, however, are most to blame. Here, the endless list includes fear of inadequacy, concern about appearance, anger, depression and feelings of worthlessness.

The able-bodied sexual partner of a disabled spouse can have just as many problems. Although some who have always considered sex distasteful are glad to end that function in their lives, many others are genuinely concerned about hurting their disabled partner during the sex act. For example, one study found that wives of heart-attack patients are almost always afraid that intercourse will cause another attack or death.[4] And when spouses find themselves repelled by changes in their disabled partner, they may withdraw from sex, give it up altogether or seek a new partner.

Most disabled individuals and their partners can be helped to resume a sexual relationship through minor adjustments in medication, frank discussion with a doctor or sexual counselling. People who want to continue the sexual aspect of their lives can usually find a way—if they are willing to try.

Some Sexual Definitions

Three terms—"sex," "sex act" and "sexuality"—are often used interchangeably, but each has a slightly different meaning. Understanding these differences helps in appreciating the sexual potential of disabled people.[5] For our purposes they can be defined as follows: *Sex* is one of four primary human drives, the others being hunger, thirst and avoidance of pain; disability eliminates none of these other drives and need not permanently damage the sex drive. A *sex act* is any physical activity involving the primary or secondary sexual organs or erogenous zones; sexual intercourse is one example of a sex act. *Sexuality* is a combination of the sex drive, sex acts and all aspects of the personality concerned with communication and relationship patterns. Conversation, shared activity, the demonstration of affection, and sexual intercourse can all be manifestations of sexuality.

Many professional counsellors contend that the *mind* is an intrinsic part of sexuality, that it is in fact the most important sex organ. Counselling based on this idea can help people change their attitudes and achieve sexual pleasure.

Attitudes About Sex

Many attitudes about sex, the sex act and sexuality prevent disabled people from enjoying their sexuality. For example, some people view the sex act as an Olympian sport with rigidly defined positions, male and female responsibilities and a finish that must include orgasm and ejaculation. If sex cannot be performed the right way, they say, it shouldn't be done at all. This narrow view turns all of human sexuality into a brief physical encounter that denies the tremendous variety in enjoyment that can exist.

Although many disabled people cannot assume standard body positions during intercourse or "cross the finish tape" every time, they do continue their sexual lives—just as some keep moving around even though they cannot walk anymore. These people have discovered these truths:

- The absence of sensation doesn't mean the absence of feeling.
- The presence of deformities doesn't mean the absence of desire.
- The inability to perform doesn't mean the inability to enjoy.
- The loss of genitals doesn't mean the loss of sexuality.[6]

Attitudes that consider sex, sex acts and sexuality as unnatural or sinful hamper sexual adjustment after disability. These attitudes include: Sex before marriage is wrong; good women do not enjoy sex; masturbation is harmful; and any sex act other than genital-to-genital contact is a perversion. All these attitudes cause incalculable guilt and anxiety; they are particularly distressing to disabled people who cannot perform within "approved guidelines" or have no sexual partner.

Attitudes—conscious or unconscious—about the purpose of the sex act also influence a couple's chances for pleasure. When sexual intercourse is viewed solely as a method of procreation, or as a means of gaining power or bestowing punishment or reward, the possibilities for enjoyment are limited. In contrast, those who see the sex act as an important form of communication, a delightful recreation and a means of reinforcing a loving relationship are more likely to find fulfillment.

Doctors are among the first to admit that they are poorly equipped to discuss patients' sexual problems.[7] Their own embarrassment, personal discomfort with sexuality, refusal to recognize the sexual needs of disabled people and lack of sexuality training all contribute to this problem. Although medical-school curricula have always included human reproduction, courses in sexuality training for medical students were almost nonexistent before 1954.[8] Only in the last

decade has sexuality of the disabled become an important subject
for medical education and research. People involved in rehabilitation now know that keeping or restoring a patient's sexual function
increases the chances for successful rehabilitation.[9]

Help With Sexual Adjustment

Although couples are influenced by a great many personal, religious and societal attitudes about sex that can cause difficulties,
their chances for resuming a sexual relationship after disability are
good if they had a happy, healthy relationship before. Couples with
rigid attitudes about sex have more trouble, especially when their
attitudes are enforced by strong religious prohibitions. And if sex
has always been a mere duty or physical act with little emotional involvement, partners probably will not want to make an adjustment.

Before seeking outside help with sexual problems, couples can
help themselves by trying to be patient and understanding. Since
the disabled partner's sexual needs continue or may even increase,
couples should try to maintain intimacy by being close and tender
and sharing expressions of love. They ought to talk about their feelings and how they can please one another. Their experiments may
eventually lead to new forms of lovemaking that place less emphasis on performance and more on enjoyment. Love, after all, is
like gift-giving; it should be as much fun to give it as to receive.

Far too many couples give up their sexual life permanently rather
than risk the embarrassment of asking for help. Some would need
only reassurance from their doctor, clergyman or counsellor that
sexual desire is normal and experimentation permissible. Others require more practical information: What activities are medically permissible, what positions are best, how to manage with equipment
the disabled partner is wearing. Although doctors are sometimes reluctant to introduce the subject of sex, they are usually willing to
discuss ranges of permissible activity and other medical aspects
when asked for help. Many physicians also recommend reading materials that help people with particular conditions, such as arthritis,
spinal cord injury or colostomy.

Doctors or medical centers can also recommend reputable sex
therapists or sex therapy clinics. The proliferation of sex therapy
clinics in this country shows that many people are concerned about
their sexual problems. For able-bodied and disabled alike, treatment
is more apt to concentrate on remolding attitudes than teaching new
techniques of prowess. When the mind is relaxed, the body enjoys.

Sex therapy has become a routine part of many rehabilitation programs, especially for patients with severely disabling conditions such as spinal cord injury. Working with their partner, patients who want to continue their sex life can usually find a way. Many, in fact, are able to have children. Contrary to popular belief, lack of orgastic ability in the woman or erectile or ejaculatory ability in the man does not indicate infertility. Therefore, couples of childbearing age with these problems who do not want to conceive should be sure to use a contraceptive method. Since some health conditions prevent women from using certain types of contraceptive, couples should consult a doctor to find a safe and effective method.

Sex and the Dying

People with terminal illness are frequently allowed to return home following hospital treatment to spend time with the family. Along with their partner, they suffer stresses compounded by fears of permanent separation. Spouses and other family members do not always recognize the dying patient's need for sexual intimacy, perhaps because they think the grief of dying and the physical deterioration leading up to death leave no room for sexual desire.

Dying patients typically go through stages in their adjustment to death, and sometimes these stages are reflected in unusual sexual behavior.[10] During the early stages, they deny the prospect of death, and may become more sexually active, even promiscuous, and may even try to conceive. When they finally admit that death is inevitable, anger sets in—often against their partner. Then as the anger turns inward, they become depressed, lose interest in sex and withdraw completely from their partner. All too often, they are emotionally isolated when death arrives.

Despite the way the dying person may be acting, there is a desperate need for affection, warmth and tenderness. Even though deeply troubled by feelings of rejection and abandonment, the partner should try to be understanding. If compassion and love can surmount these feelings, the sharing of intimate pleasures can make the closing months of life more bearable for both patient and surviving spouse.

Disabled People Without Partners

Disabled individuals who have no sexual partner can be in particularly desperate straits because they have no one who is very close to bolster their sexual self-esteem. Since sexuality can take many forms, however, these people should be encouraged to participate in social activities to develop new relationships and ways to express sexuality. In addition, they should be given privacy to satisfy their needs through masturbation. Above all, we must respect them as normal, sexual human beings worthy and capable of receiving pleasure and giving happiness to another person.

A meaningful sexual relationship, then, helps to rebuild self-confidence. To assume that every disabled person can have an active sex life is perhaps too optimistic, but to decide that sex is not important for a particular individual, simply because he is disabled, is destructive. The emphasis given here to sex is not to suggest that it ought to be the only activity to fill the boring hours of convalescence; rather, that its importance must be recognized and promoted.

FAMILY RELATIONSHIPS

The immediate family forms the next circle, after that of the spouse, around the disabled person. Just as it does with sexual relationships, disability disrupts and causes problems with family relationships. Some families weather the storm while others are torn apart. However stable the family, the impact of disability can swamp it. Family members must work together, swap tasks and spell one another if they want to stay afloat and save all hands.

Too often, families unwittingly allow the effects of disability to spread far beyond their relative's actual limitations. Fathers who lose their jobs are deprived of all family respect and authority, mothers who can no longer care for their homes are relieved of all mothering duties, and grandparents and mature children who must give up independent living are relegated to childlike roles.

The disabled person is greatly affected by the way in which his family receives him back into the home. Pampering and overprotection or isolation will strip him of all his remaining self-respect. But if he is accepted as a still-valuable part of the family who must be involved in decisions and workload, he will feel strong. The prestige he gains from being important to his family will carry over into other relationships in his life.

Families can use the convalescent period, then, to help the patient adjust to his disability and prepare to resume a nearly normal, although probably different, life. Three areas in which they can have the most influence are his self-care and independence, involvement in the family, and personal development.

Encouraging Self-Care and Independence

The desire to pamper the patient can lead us to do everything for him, deciding even what he wears, when he eats and how he spends his time. But even when he cannot attend to his own needs, he must decide how and when his family will help him. We can suggest, but he ought to be the boss. Less restricted individuals must be encouraged to assume maximum responsibility for their personal care and treatment. Patients on special diets, for example, can read about foods and recipes, and help with menu planning, grocery shopping and food preparation. We can give someone learning to administer insulin to himself or care for a new colostomy a storage area for supplies and responsibility for its maintenance. Instead of fussing over and waiting on him, we must insist that our relative do for himself. At times like this, a sense of humor is invaluable.

> When Lisa first came home from the hospital, she wore a metal head frame and full casts on one arm and both legs. All this equipment, plus a broken collarbone that grated whenever she moved, severely restricted her mobility. Although we placed every possible convenience within reach of her unencumbered hand, insisting that she fend for herself, she still needed a great deal of help. To relieve her distress at being so dependent, I began to call her "Fairy Princess"—the one upon whom we all must wait.
>
> "So, the Fairy Princess needs a bedpan! Can't she get it herself?" I would say. Or, "Don't tell me the Fairy Princess needs help getting into her wheelchair again!" Goaded by humor, Lisa spent hours plotting her revenge.
>
> Then when we did offer help, she would suddenly announce in a regal tone, "The Fairy Princess doesn't need your help with *that* anymore!" As she struggled with some simple task, we would helplessly stand by, watching the perspiration spill from her forehead. Finally, exhausted but triumphant, she would look up and ask, "How many fairy princesses do you know who can do that?"

It is tempting to wait on the patient because it feels good to be needed and it is painful to see him struggle. It is much easier to make decisions and do things quickly ourselves—besides, we have other work to do. But making him feel dependent in his own household deprives him of countless opportunities to be successful. He will never learn to feel good about himself.

Another concern during convalescence is clothing, for two reasons. First, because looking good makes a person feel good; second, because the ability to dress oneself encourages independence. Disabled, sick or deformed people often lose interest in their appearance. Since they have few contacts with other people during convalescence, many prefer to wear bedclothes or comfortable but unattractive clothing. We ought to encourage our relative to dress up a bit and spend some time on personal grooming; and when he does make the effort, we should be ready with compliments.

Clothing ought to be attractive but functional; fabrics should be easy to care for and strong but not bulky; fastenings should be conveniently placed and easy to operate; and garment design should be comfortable and unrestrictive.[11] Minor garment adjustments often help a person dress himself. People who are severely deformed or confined to a wheelchair require more extensive clothing alterations. Several sources supply patterns, alteration instructions and adaptive clothing.* If need be, clever friends or a local seamstress can help with sewing.

Our disabled relative will also feel more independent if we remove obstacles that impede his movement and ability to function in the home. Home modifications are especially important if his disability is permanent. Many people gain a great amount of freedom through very simple changes such as replacement of light switches, door knobs or faucets. For someone who uses a wheelchair more extensive alterations may be needed: widening doorways, altering a kitchen or bathroom or building ramps over stairs. Innumerable books and brochures suggest home modifications that range from the ridiculously simple to the sublimely complex.† Hospital occupational therapists can help solve particular problems of living arrangements. Financial assistance for modifications is often available, regardless of income, from the federal Department of Housing and Urban Development through municipal or county social-service ("welfare") departments.

When a disabled person realizes that his family is willing to modify his clothing and home environment so that he can function independently, he starts to seek his own solutions for overcoming his handicaps. He begins to think about *how,* not *if,* he can manage with his disability.

---

* Some of these, including a glove and shoe exchange for amputees, are listed in Appendix B under "Personal Care: Clothing and Living Aids."
† Appendix B lists these resources under "Housing and Home Services."

Encouraging Involvement in the Family

Families tend to shield a convalescing disabled perso
lems caused by his presence in the household. Althoug
tions are kind, they ought to instead include h
deliberations, because their problems concern him as much as the
rest of the family. Despite his disability, he may be willing and able
to make sacrifices that help solve these problems.

> Grandma Marshall had to stay with her son's family for several
> weeks after her surgery. Nobody expected any problems because
> the family had a spare room and her daughter-in-law was glad to
> care for her. However, the family's teenagers clearly resented
> Grandma's presence; she disliked their noise and her needs made
> their mother too busy to cater to some of theirs.
>
> Grandma's son and daughter-in-law were tempted to scold
> their children for being selfish, but knew that their resentment
> would only have grown. Instead, they included Grandma in their
> discussions. When she learned that her dislike of the children's
> noise was so obvious, she offered to retreat to her room when their
> activities became too loud for her; and she suggested ways she
> could help her daughter-in-law with household tasks. She was
> happy to do all these things, she said, to repay her family for their
> hospitality.
>
> Everyone was relieved when Grandma finally was able to return
> to her own apartment. Her stay had been a valuable experience,
> however; the children learned about cooperation and gained a
> new respect for their grandmother; she, in turn, was proud of her
> role in solving the crisis and her elevated status in the family.

People who are convalescing need periods of privacy and restful
quiet, but large doses of isolation are lethal. Whenever possible,
they should be included in family meals and other activities. Even
when they cannot actively participate in what the family is doing,
they get pleasure simply from being involved.

Finally, we must help our relative to keep his old role in the family or assign him a new one suitable to his abilities. If a mother must
become the breadwinner when her husband is disabled, for example, she need not take over all the chores of being both mother and
father. Regardless of his limitations, her husband usually can continue to perform some of his fatherly duties and learn other household jobs. Although deprived of his breadwinning role, he will
regain self-respect when he finds he can still contribute to the family enterprise, albeit in a different way. Rearranging family duties

ᵢten seems to take more time than it's worth, but helping a relative feel useful is an invaluable gift.

Encouraging Personal Development

Filling the empty days of convalescence means more than being a recreational director. Although we aim to please and amuse, we should use this time to help our relative develop new interests and put his skills to work. Any activity that captures his interest and imagination will serve this purpose; when the activity is channelled into service for others, the results are far more rewarding.

> Mr. Bush had been employed by an electrical firm before an accident made him a paraplegic. While he was convalescing at home, his inactivity and constant diet of television brought him to the brink of severe depression. Finally, his wife asked him to repair some long-neglected small appliances. His success with these prompted him to place an announcement in his church bulletin, offering to make repairs for senior citizens for the cost of parts. A store owner, hearing of his project, offered him a discount on parts. Filled with a sense of purpose and pride, Mr. Bush was ready far sooner than expected for job retraining by his firm.

> Mrs. Carlton was active in local politics until reconstructive surgery for arthritis threatened to sideline her during a local election. Her husband offered their home to a local candidate to use as his campaign headquarters so she could remain in the midst of campaign activity.

In other instances, a disabled mother's family collected yarn from friends so she could knit mittens for their church bazaar; a convalescing man learned to back cookies, and soon attracted a huge following of young neighbors who helped with the baking and consumption of his products; and a man who had to forgo his large vegetable garden one spring put his green thumb to work raising house plants for residents in a nearby nursing home.

The convalescing person who cannot perform his customary activities and has too much time on his hands is apt to think only about himself. If his thoughts and skills are channelled into worthwhile projects, he gains a tremendous sense of accomplishment. Everyone, no matter how physically disabled, has some ability he can share with others. Our task is to find it and put it to work.

Books, records and radio and television programs all provide opportunities for personal enrichment as well as entertainment. Many services help to make these resources more accessible to disabled people. For example, public libraries offer to the visually impaired a variety of tapes, records and large-print books. When these items are not available locally, librarians can obtain them, usually free of charge, through interlibrary loan programs.

The Library of Congress Talking Book Service for the Blind and Physically Handicapped provides recorded materials to anyone with a temporary or permanent visual, physical or reading impairment—in other words, anyone who has trouble reading. Each subscriber is supplied with special slow-speed equipment and voluminous catalogs of listening materials. All this is free. Public libraries have application forms for this service. Choice Magazine Listening, a non-profit organization, sends listening materials to its subscribers free of charge. These include bimonthly recordings of unabridged articles from such publications as *Smithsonian, Saturday Review, Sports Illustrated* and *Playboy.*

The Library of Congress also has music services—including recordings and large-print and braille music—and catalogs of communication aids and appliances and adaptive equipment for the blind and physically handicapped. These materials can be ordered through local libraries or from the Library of Congress in Washington, D.C.

More than 100 radio stations across the country now provide a radio information and reading service for people who cannot read. They supply free program guides and a decoding device which allows people to hear a wide range of programs, including news and entertainment features. Much of the programming is prepared by National Public Radio's Service for the Print Handicapped. Public libraries, state public radio stations and National Public Radio in Washington, D.C. provide information about local radio stations that supply this service. Due to limited funds, some areas have a waiting list for receiving devices; however, individuals can sometimes purchase their own at a nominal cost.

For people with hearing impairments, electronics stores sell amplification devices for radio and television sets. In addition, Sears, Roebuck and Co. sells telecaption adapters, devices that permit the viewer to see a subtitled transcription of the audio portion of television programming at the bottom of the screen.

Correspondence courses can be fun and profitable for the person who faces a long convalescence; they can be used in developing new skills, beginning a new career or continuing a disrupted education.

Schools offer literally hundreds of courses on every conceivable subject for personal enrichment or credit towards a diploma and degree. However, since many service providers have entered this field to take money from the unsuspecting, it is best to investigate before enrollment. Local high school or college guidance counsellors can be a good resource here. In addition, the National Home Study Commission supplies free copies of their *Directory of Accredited Home Study Schools* with a listing of courses.*

When someone has a permanent disability, he can use convalescent time to learn how others have coped with similar circumstances. Despite all the information he may have received from his doctor and other health care providers, he is likely to have many more questions after hospital discharge. Organizations dedicated to serving people with disabling conditions of every type abound. They provide informative publications, regular newsletters and referral services. Local chapters offer support services through self-help groups. Public health nurses can also help to locate self-help groups.

During convalescence, then, we are in an ideal position to help our relative use time productively. Our efforts to encourage independence, involvement in family affairs and personal development can greatly improve his chances for successful adjustment to disability.

RELATIONSHIPS WITH FRIENDS

Disability can destroy a friendship. Often the disabled person can no longer participate in the shared activities that bind friendships together. He may find that some people have trouble relating to a disabled friend when pity contaminates their relationship: They become guarded; for fear of offending, they avoid common, everyday words that have suddenly taken on new significance. On the other hand, a disabled person may be so preoccupied with his problems that he is no longer good company.

Friends who were attentive at first may abandon a disabled person during convalescence, because they become increasingly uncomfortable or simply bored when around him. Even when they try to maintain their friendship, their very presence reminds their disabled friend of all that he has lost. He feels worthless because they are nicely dressed while he is wearing a robe or old clothes, they can

* See "Employment and Education" in Appendix B.

talk well while he must grope for words or they are busy while he is not.

Family members are expected to provide a disabled person with love and security; if they fail in this, the whole family is likely to suffer the consequences. Friends have no such obligation; they are free to make the effort or not as they choose. They have their own lives to lead and can easily find others with whom to share activities.

As friends of a disabled person, our help is particularly valuable because we *choose* to give it. When we make the effort to be with him and treat him as formerly, we convince him of his continuing value. When we accept him, he sees the possibility that others will treat him as a person rather than an object to be avoided. On the other hand, rejection, insincerity or profuse demonstrations of pity force him to assume that he will encounter similar behavior from everyone he meets. "If my friends treat me this way," he reasons, "how can I expect better treatment from other people?"

Special Hints for Friends

Although most convalescing people are delighted by surprise visits that break the monotony of their days, visits are best scheduled in advance, unless they are frequent and regular. This courtesy gives the patient a chance to prepare for the visit and enjoy the anticipation of its diversion. Every effort should be made to keep the arrangements. Cancellations of plans with friends are always disappointing; during convalescence, they are devastating because they reinforce feelings of worthlessness.

Whenever possible, it is a good idea to plan a visit around an activity or project—something that will divert the disabled person's attention from his disability and remind him that he can still participate in shared interests. The involvement of other people—perhaps a small group of friends to play cards or watch a television show— can also give him a chance to participate in group activities in the security of his home. Especially in cases of severe disability or deformity, a person needs to feel comfortable relating to friends in his own home before he can face them in other situations.

We ought to encourage our disabled friend to take part in previously shared activities outside his home, even when his participation must be at a different level. By enlisting a former athletic team member to help with coaching, for example, we can maintain his interest and help him feel valuable.

Activities with disabled friends should be planned to minimize limitations. A person who has lost an arm can manage picnic fare, but may feel uncomfortable in a restaurant where someone has to cut his meat. An outdoor movie theatre makes a handicap less obvious than an indoor one, where parking, curbs, doors, stairs and seating have to be negotiated. Whatever the circumstance, it is important to let a disabled person do as much as he can for himself; he may need help getting into a restaurant, for example, but he can still choose where and what he wants to eat.

Knowing how to offer assistance without making a disabled person feel helpless and inferior is difficult.[12] Sometimes we only learn that skill by making many embarrassing mistakes. In most cases, it is best to ask permission and wait to be told how to help: "Can I help you into the car, or can you manage on your own?" When a disabled friend wants to do things on his own, we should allow him the extra time needed. Praise should be sincere—showing that we recognize his effort—but not effusive.

For some of us, conversation with a disabled person is another problem.[13] Our reaction to his condition—perhaps a cancerous tumor or disfigurement—can make small talk seem impossible. In this situation, we should force ourselves to concentrate on subjects that interest him—sports, current events, family activities—anything that will keep the conversation going. If he chooses to discuss his condition, we ought to listen sympathetically and encourage him to express his feelings, without prying to satisfy our own curiosity. If he has a speech problem that involves faltering, the temptation to guess what he wants to say and complete his sentences for him is natural; we want him to hurry up and finish so we can respond. This, of course, is not helpful; we must be patient. By pacing conversations more slowly, we give him time to express himself and prevent unnecessary frustration.

Learning how to relate to a disabled friend is fraught with difficulty. Regardless of the circumstances, we will do much better if we forget his disability and concentrate on him as a friend. He will forgive our bumbling mistakes because he values our friendship.

THE OUTER CIRCLE:
ACQUAINTANCES AND STRANGERS

All of us remember from childhood encountering a disabled person, one we recognized as being different from other people. Just as we were pointing and beginning to ask, "Mommy, why does that lady . . . ?" mother yanked us on the arm, silenced us with a hand over the mouth and dragged us quickly from the scene.

Every relationship in an individual's life is disturbed when he is obviously disabled. Ordinary transactions, with friends or strangers, are different. Children stare and adults look with pity or avoid eye contact altogether. People assume that the disabled person can do nothing for himself. "What does she take in her coffee?" a waitress asks the husband whose wife uses a wheelchair. Or, worse still, they smother the handicapped person with a heavy cloud of obvious and embarrassing attention.

Facing the world with a disability can be so terrifying that some people vow never to leave the security of home. We cannot protect our disabled relative or friend from all the unthinking people he is likely to meet, but we can help him develop some self-assurance and a thick skin. To make his initial trips out into the community as comfortable as possible, we can help him choose situations where he will feel at ease and from which he can leave at will.

We can also join the campaign for the acceptance of disabled people by refusing to accept rude or overly attentive behavior. We might say, "It's alright for your child to be curious—that's a good way for him to learn about disabled people," "Why don't you ask my wife what she wants in her coffee?" or "You needn't bother helping him; he can manage for himself." When we teach others that disability does not devalue someone as a human being, the disabled person learns that lesson, too.

As one successful experience outside his home builds on another, he gains the courage to try more challenging situations. Finally, he will be so proud of himself he wants to shout to anyone who will listen, "I may be disabled, but I'd like to see *you* do half as well in my shoes!"

CHAPTER 5

Help for the Helpers

DISABILITY OFTEN AFFECTS THE REST OF US in the family as decisively as our sick or injured relative. Even though troubled by all sorts of new worries and responsibilities, we think we are supposed to be brave and strong. With all our concern focussed on the patient, we may not realize—or be willing to admit—that we, the helpers, need as much help as he does.

Most of us do need help when caring for or living with a disabled person. In fact, some of us need help even before bringing him home from the hospital. The extraordinary stress of disability can seriously threaten our relationship with the patient and our own personal well-being.

We will start by looking at the ways in which disability causes stress in the family and how that stress can affect everyone's health and behavior. After that, we will look at a few ways for managing this new stress in our lives.

CAUSES AND SIGNS OF STRESS

Stress is really a condition of life. Only death relieves an individual of all stress. Although we have little control over most of the stress we encounter in life, we do have a choice in how to cope with it. We can regard emotional stress as an opportunity for personal growth, just as an athlete uses physical stress to strengthen his body. Successfully coping with a stressful event gives us new abilities and a sense of accomplishment. On the other hand, we can let stress abuse us, so that we feel helpless and anxious.

Any change in our normal living patterns will cause stress, whether we regard that change as a happy or unhappy event. For example, changes in marital or job status are stressful for both the directly affected person and his family. Two psychiatrists at the University of Washington Medical School have devised a Social Readjustment Scale which identifies and measures major stressful life events. This scale includes changes in the health of a family member, financial status, work responsibilities, living conditions, recreation patterns and social activities, as well as eating, sleeping and sexual habits.[1] These changes can occur when a family member becomes disabled; they cause stress because they threaten our personal security and accustomed patterns of living.

The body's reaction to any threat is automatic and beyond the individual's control. Sensing a real or imagined danger, the brain sends signals to the glands and nervous system, activating a series of bodily responses. A person frightened by an intruder in his home feels these responses. His heart pounds in his chest as he begins to perspire and breathe faster. Without any conscious direction from the mind, his body is preparing to react to danger. Within seconds he is ready to either fight off the intruder or flee with dispatch through the nearest exit. Whatever his choice, he seems to possess almost superhuman speed and strength.

This automatic emergency response—the "fight-or-flight response"—is the same response we experience when confronted by the very real threats associated with disability. The loss of security and changes in our living patterns and plans for the future—all are as great a threat to personal well-being as the intruder entering the home.

Faced with the threats that disability presents, we can choose to fight by attacking what seems the cause of our problem. We can fight with our disabled relative, because we blame him for his and our misfortune. We can fight with the rest of the family, with medical personnel, with others who we feel are responsible for his condition. We can even fight with ourselves because we feel somehow at fault.

Or we can flee. We can abandon or ignore our relative. We can resort to pills, alcohol or other drugs for escape, or withdraw emotionally or physically from our responsibilities. We can unconsciously develop our own illness which prevents us from caring for him or performing other tasks. Researchers have found that when one family member becomes chronically disabled, other family members often develop symptoms that relieve them of responsibility and divert attention away from the original patient. Sometimes, in fact, a spouse shows more symptoms than his or her disabled partner.[2]

The desire to fight or flee is a profoundly normal reaction to the threats associated with disability. Most forms of fighting, however, are inappropriate and unproductive in this context. Fleeing brings temporary relief, but does nothing to resolve the crisis. As much as we would like to fight or flee, most of us try to avoid such behavior because we realize it will not solve our problems and could make things even worse.

Instead, we resort to a third alternative: simply to wait fearfully. We cower like a trapped animal who knows it is no match for its enemy yet sees no route for escape. Trapped by all our problems, we wait helplessly for some outside force to come along and decide our fate. Waiting to see what will happen, we are paralyzed by anxiety.

Quite simply, anxiety is the internalization of the fight-or-flight response—a turning inward of fears. Still sensing danger, the brain continues to send signals to the body: "Prepare to fight or flee. Keep the heart pumping. Keep the blood pressure up. Maintain all systems at top speed." Constantly bombarded by emotional and physical warning signals, we experience stress.

In small doses, stress can be a catalyst for personal growth if it forces us to broaden our horizons and seek new solutions to problems. Unrelieved stress, however, is unhealthy. When the body and mind are constantly forced to work overtime we become mentally and physically exhausted. We nag and cry; tempers flare. We lose appetite or overeat; suffer from diarrhea or constipation; sleep all the time or not at all; are restless or lethargic. Carried to extremes, we may develop heart disease, hypertension, chronic bowel problems, allergies, skin disorders, ulcers or mental illness.

Most of us are unlikely to develop extreme manifestations of stress unless our problems are long-standing and unresolved. But we are likely to show such telltale signs of stress as fatigue, irritability and sleeplessness. We may ignore these symptoms, perhaps because we feel guilty thinking about ourselves, or we may accept them as an inevitable consequence of our situation. However much we try to suffer in silence, everyone around will be affected.

We can learn to cope with stress in "three easy steps." First, we must learn to recognize and express our feelings, dealing with them out in the open rather than letting them fester within and cause more stress. Second, we must find healthy outlets for fight-and-flight responses, and protect our bodies from the damaging side effects of stress. Third, we should change and control our environment if necessary, to rid ourselves of some of the causes of stress. In varying degrees, all three of these suggestions call for courage—that is, a conscious effort to overcome difficult problems. Courage is, after all, not the absence of fear, but the ability to move ahead even when we are afraid.[3]

Disability in our family tends to inspire feelings of fear, anger, frustration, guilt and depression. All of these feelings are normal, but their focus is not always appropriate. For example, anger is appropriate when directed towards a drunken driver who has maimed a relative, or an employer whose negligence has caused the injury of a loved one. On the other hand, anger is inappropriate when we think, "I'm mad at her because she has cancer and has spoiled my plans for retirement." Similarly, sadness is appropriate when someone we love is disabled, but depression is inappropriate if we blame ourselves unrealistically for his condition: "My husband wouldn't have had his heart attack if I had insisted he eat the right foods."

When involved in caring for a disabled relative, we experience many inappropriate feelings: "I'm the only one who can care for him," "He's totally dependent on me for his care and his feelings would be hurt if I abandoned him for even a few hours," "People expect me to sacrifice everything for him; his disability is my new lot in life," "I must be at fault and I have to pay the consequences," "The only way to get everything done is to work constantly and worry the rest of the time."

All these feelings represent repressed anger at threats to personal security, anger turned inward because we cannot bear to express it to ourselves or anyone else. We feel guilty. We become depressed and feel the need to suffer, to punish ourselves. Although depression is a normal form of hurting, it is a profound and shattering hurt.

In his *Choices: Coping Creatively With Personal Change*, psychiatrist Frederic Flack describes depression as "a falling apart." However, he says that depression is a "necessary part of the creative and healing process," pointing out that most people who become depressed recover in time. We tend to admire people who remain calm under pressure, and to view fear and depression as weaknesses. But Dr. Flack reports that when people do not allow themselves to "fall apart" and recover, they expend most of their energy holding themselves together in one piece. Although they may appear to be calm, they experience a crippling spiritual and emotional corrosion.[4]

In order to constructively fall apart, we have to admit and express our feelings. This expression of feelings can take many forms, including outbursts of rage and crying. However, most people find that simply talking to someone who tries to understand without passing judgment is a far more helpful form of relief. Close friends who are good listeners are invaluable in this regard, because they provide a sounding board on which we can vent our anger and frustration. Further, they can help by discouraging inappropriate thoughts: "Now, Mary, be sensible. You know very well you couldn't do anything to change John's eating habits. You're not responsible for his heart attack," or, "Don, I know you're angry because Joan's cancer has disrupted all your plans, but that's not her fault!" Our friends can give us new perspectives, point out our strengths and help us search for solutions when we feel helpless.

Those of us with such friends are lucky. Their love and patience permit us to say what we feel; their common sense helps us reevaluate feelings and circumstances. If we have no close friends who can give this kind of help, or if our problems seem overwhelming, we ought to consider finding someone else, perhaps a professional counsellor, to help.

Some of the danger signals that point to a need for professional counselling include persistent feelings of frustration, irritability, annoyance, anger, guilt or depression.

Professional counselling can also help us to deal with our relative's feelings. Many families fail to realize that disability can cause the patient to behave abnormally. For example, they may react to his outbursts of anger as personal attacks, when in reality he has no control over his behavior. We ought to seek advice, then, if we have problems relating to our disabled relative because he is depressed, overly dependent, impatient, irritable or has severe mood changes.

We may also need professional help if we are deeply troubled by a lack of social contact, financial worries, or problems in coping with new responsibilities.

Fortunately, we have many places to turn to for help. While our relative is hospitalized or receiving out-patient treatment, we can ask to meet with counsellors in the hospital's rehabilitation, social service or pastoral care departments. At other times, our resources include community mental health agencies, public and private (often religiously affiliated) social-service agencies, the clergy and self-help groups. Doctors and nurses, chambers of commerce, United Way offices and public libraries should all be familiar with mental health resources in their community.

No one should feel shamed by the need for professional counselling when upset. Rather than a sign of weakness, the ability to constructively "fall apart" shows we have the courage to face our feelings. To return to Dr. Flack once more:

> The majority of people who have consulted me over the years seem healthier than many others I have encountered outside the consulting room. The others, lacking insight, unmotivated to improve, blaming their problems on the people around them, rarely if ever seek professional help. Working things out, to them, always depends on someone else's changing.[5]

Friends and professional counsellors are important sources of emotional relief. Often we can talk more easily with outsiders; we fear we will hurt those we love if we tell them how angry we are with them. Nevertheless, we must maintain—or develop—honest communication among family members in the difficult circumstances of disability. We can set an example by being honest about our own feelings. If we feel overworked: "I'm angry because I seem to be doing all the work around here. What can you do to help me?" Or to a disabled relative who is overly demanding: "I'm upset because you call me all the time. You're not doing as much as you can for yourself." Others will be temporarily hurt by our outbursts, but they will be able to handle them (and possibly help relieve our distress) because we have given them the reason for our anger. In contrast, hostile and resentful behavior, caused by hidden anger, is bewildering, destructive and impossible to deal with. Everyone will be better off, then, if we get things off our chest and clear the air when upset—and encourage other family members to do the same.

Physical exercise relieves stress. It uses up the pressures of fight-or-flight responses and is a tremendous outlet for feelings. Slamming a door or pounding a fist on a table rapidly dispels anger; sports or activities requiring strenuous physical exertion are just as effective, but more enjoyable. A trite but true prescription: Regular exercise combined with proper diet and adequate rest will protect us from the ravages of stress and revive our stamina.

Many medical authorities also recommend regular use of relaxation techniques to combat stress. The methods, including yoga and Transcendental Meditation, have common elements: a quiet environment, a comfortable position and concentration on pleasant thoughts to the exclusion of all others. We can easily adapt these elements to our circumstances by taking time out each day for some form of self-indulgent relaxation, be it quiet contemplation, reading, a nap or a soothing warm bath.

Family social activities and recreation are often disrupted or curtailed when a relative becomes disabled. Family members may have too many new duties or feel guilty about having fun when one of their own is incapacitated or suffering. However, regardless of how pressed for time or guilty they may feel, each family member should set aside recreation time. Recreation—any diversion from routine and responsibilities—is an excellent release valve for stress, one that is vitally important to mental health.

When trying to cope with caring for a disabled person, we *know* there is no time in the day for trivial exercise, relaxation or recreation; every minute is filled with extra tasks and our disabled relative's care. But wait: Even though we feel guilty thinking of ourselves, each of us has important needs that should not be ignored. Especially when no one else is concentrating on our welfare, we must learn to say, "I want some time for myself. I need to get away for a while. I love you, but I have to love myself, too." By taking the time to please ourselves, we invariably become more pleasant to live with.

REDUCING CAUSES OF STRESS

Coping with stress involves controlling the *causes*, as well as the *effects*, of stress. In order to do this we must identify our problems. Then comes the hard part: deciding which problems can be solved and which are beyond our control.

Many families feel powerless to solve their problems; thinking they are helpless, they develop anxiety and stress building to intolerable limits. For this very reason, families with severely and chronically disabled relatives suffer an exceptionally high rate of breakdown.[6] We must be convinced, then, that we have the ability to solve our problems; if we feel powerless, we will be.

When a relative is disabled, we obviously have no control over the primary cause of stress—that is, his disability. We can reduce his handicap by ensuring proper treatment and rehabilitation, but the fact of accident or disease is immutable. We can, however, reduce other causes of stress that result from the disability. Such a cause is lack of confidence in our ability to render proper care. We can significantly reduce this apprehension by learning all we need to know about our relative's condition and treatment. Doctors, nurses and rehabilitation staff are available to answer questions during hospitalization, but they can also be called upon to help with any problems encountered at home. Their help is as close as the telephone. In addition, they can refer us to public-health or visiting nurses for instruction in managing care and coping with emergencies. When we know what to expect and how to act, we will feel in control, and stress will diminish.

Self-help groups are another valuable resource in this regard. Disabled people and their families in these groups have had first-hand experience with the same problems that concern us. By joining one of these groups, we can profit from their experiences and gain support. Anyone who has learned to deal with a similar disability can be of help; invariably these people are proud of their accomplishments and eager to share their solutions.

Even when we feel prepared to cope with the details of the patient's care, we are apt to be overwhelmed by all the new responsibilities—especially if we have other commitments to job and family. It is easy to feel, as we scramble through each day, that there is no time even to think. However, if we want to control stress, we *must* take time out to think. In examining our duties, we will find that some of them are more important than others. Very often this assessment of priorities demands a change in values. A father who has been active in business and community affairs, for example, may have to reduce the value he places on community involvement when his wife becomes disabled and he is needed at home. Similarly a mother who prides herself on her ability to maintain a spotless home and cook fancy family meals every night may have to devalue these homemaking jobs when a member of her family develops more pressing needs. She must learn that she cannot do everything. She should try to do what is important and forget the rest.

Setting priorities is just the first step. The next is to enlist the help of other people, wherever and whenever we can find them:

• other family members to help with household jobs
  and the patient's care

- visiting nurses and home health aides to assist with nursing care
- relatives and friends to stay with the patient so we have time for other activities
- community day-care and other respite services for temporary relief from caregiving duties
- home-delivered meals and other home services for the disabled and elderly
- church groups and community organizations for transportation and other services
- part-time or live-in help when sufficient money is available

Involving other people in our relative's care has many advantages besides the obvious relief gained. For example, some disabled people are more comfortable when professional or paraprofessional outsiders help with details of their personal care. Professionals also can give adequate medical supervision and ensure that our attitudes about the patient and his condition remain objective. When we recruit friends and other relatives, we give them a chance to demonstrate their concern and to continue their relationship with the disabled person. Finally, and most significant, he will enjoy the diversion of having others around, and will reap the benefits of our relaxed attitudes when we feel rested.

Earlier we noted that many forms of fighting are inappropriate, because they do nothing to solve a problem or reduce stress. Fighting can be very productive, however, when we direct our energies constructively towards situations that we can change. For example, we can dispute employers' or insurance companies' decisions when we feel they are unjustly withholding benefits. We can doggedly insist that our disabled relative receive services that are being withheld due to bureaucratic red tape and fumbling. We can do battle with people who fail to observe the legal rights of disabled people. Polite and assertive fighting is highly satisfying because it can be very effective.

> When Lisa was injured, our family suffered a great deal of stress. The emotional hurt of her disfigurement and her need for support were difficult for all of us to handle, even with the generous support of friends. Ultimately, I "fell apart" under the strain and sought professional counselling. As it turned out, this was an enormous advantage to me as well as the rest of my family; we learned to cope with all the feelings brought on by Lisa's disability. We still

had to deal with many episodes of anger, guilt, resentment, jealousy and depression, but our understanding of their cause made life easier.

During Lisa's hospitalization, I spent much of each day with her, to the exclusion of all other obligations. As difficult as those days were, I suspected that I would face far greater pressures when we took her home. Her relative helplessness and great need for attention were bound to tax the limits of my endurance. To protect myself, I began to make plans even before Lisa was discharged from the hospital. Public health nurses helped me to find a variety of sickroom items that would make her care easier. After much searching, I finally located, through a hospital employment office, a licensed practical nurse who was willing to help several mornings each week with Lisa's nursing care. On inquiry, I learned that our health insurance policy and Lisa's automobile insurance policy would cover charges for her sickroom equipment and nurse. Once she came home, I gratefully accepted the offers of family and friends to help with household chores and keep Lisa company when I needed free time.

At first, Lisa viewed my eagerness to engage others in her care as a lack of love and concern. She complained about the way other people cared for her, even though they followed my careful instructions. I could have pleased her only by remaining constantly in attendance. Had I agreed to her unspoken demands, I would have collapsed from fatigue and resentment. She finally came to accept my need for help, but, more important, she became motivated to do more for herself in order not to have to rely on other people for her care.

Lisa's emotional and physical recovery were my greatest priorities during that time, but I recognized that the rest of us also had needs that deserved attention. When I got help with her care, I often squandered my free time doing special favors for my other two children and my husband or simply having fun with friends. I neglected my household and community obligations, though not without some guilt. But I felt good because I managed to stay fairly relaxed and keep some vestiges of my sense of humor. Had I not received help, I would have been worthless to myself and my family.

Some people are willing to endure exceptionally high levels of emotional stress and crushing work loads because they think that needing help is a sign of weakness. However, unless we want to be martyrs, most of us can use help in caring for a disabled family member. We help ourselves and the disabled person when we rely on others.

After everything has been said about coping with the stress of disability, perhaps the best prescription lies in Reinhold Niebuhr's well-known and immensely practical prayer:[7]

God give us grace to accept with serenity the things that cannot be changed, courage to change the things which should be changed and the wisdom to distinguish the one from the other.

CHAPTER 6

Getting Back Into the Real World

THE "REAL WORLD" IS DESIGNED for able-bodied people who can move about freely for work or play. The disabled are often locked out of that world by all sorts of barriers. Some mentally alert and intelligent individuals, for example, are shut away in institutions because they need help with their personal care; others, hardly less isolated, are barricaded in their homes because they lack transportation, employment or recreational opportunities.

The job of helping a disabled person get back into the real world involves destroying the barriers that keep him out. Rather than trying to change an "abnormal" person to fit into a "normal" environment, we have to change the environment to fit anyone who wants to lead a productive life in his community. Since invisible barriers of ignorance and prejudice are far more difficult to overcome than the obvious physical obstacles that disabled people encounter, this job calls for a large supply of gritty determination.

Many disabled people do not try to be self-sufficient because they are happy to be dependent, or they think they have no choice but to be. Their own attitudes are more confining than any external obstacles. Such individuals must be encouraged to expect more from life than a dreary day-to-day existence.

Even when a disabled family member is eager to return to a normal life in his community, doing so still requires tremendous amounts of perseverance. Most people who are trying to breach the barricades give up after a few unsuccessful attempts. In some instances, they eventually succeed only because the family is willing to withstand considerable difficulty on their behalf. Like them, we will encounter many people who place our telephone calls on indefinite hold, deny without reason our requests for help or shuffle us from one agency to another. All these indignities are bearable only if we are convinced that through persistence we can help our relative succeed.

The barriers that keep disabled people from leading normal lives involve problems associated with personal care and supervision, housing, transportation, architectural access, employment, education, recreation and travel. In this chapter, we will first look at some solutions to these particular problems and then at some possibilities for legal and group action.*

PERSONAL CARE AND SUPERVISION

Disabled people are often forced into institutions because they cannot care for themselves. However, these individuals can sometimes function quite independently in other areas of life, when given a chance. Many elderly people, for example, are able to stay in the community and out of the nursing home because their family and friends provide them with daily visits, telephone calls, meals and chore assistance. In fact, many quadriplegics and others with total physical disability lead productive lives with the help of full-time personal attendants.

Before consigning a relative to a nursing home or other institution, we ought to examine carefully his personal needs to see if he could possibly manage at home with outside help. If we cannot help him ourselves, public health nurses or social workers can assist in locating necessary services—visiting nurses, home health aides, homemakers or home-delivered meals, perhaps. Often these simple but vital services allow people to remain at home, close to their regular activities and friends. Fees for these services are usually based on

* A listing of organizations and other resources that pertain to the topics covered in this chapter appears in the back matter as "Appendix B: Organizations Providing Specific Types of Services."

ability to pay, or may be covered, in instances of *skilled* health care, by a health insurance policy.

Finding a personal attendant or someone to provide continuous supervision for a disabled person is far more difficult. Large city employment agencies often supply attendant care, but their charges are too high for most budgets. Possible sources of less costly full- or part-time help include elderly residents living in housing developments, senior citizen organizations, high school or college student employment offices, nursing schools, agencies that serve the mildly retarded and housewives. Classified ads, church newsletters or community bulletin boards also can produce results.

Chances of finding a suitable attendant improve when we can appropriately match the age, sex and needs of our disabled relative with the qualifications and needs of prospective employees. For example, elderly citizens who want to supplement their Social Security income manage well in caring for someone their own age, if care requirements are not strenuous. Students who need housing and pocket money are ideal attendants for the person who wants young, part-time help. Mildly retarded individuals can make excellent attendants when tasks are repetitive or guidance is readily available.

Since attendants are ultimately responsible to the disabled person, he should be involved in every aspect of the hiring process, unless he is mentally impaired. Once a prospective candidate is located, our relative should conduct the interviews, decide whom he will hire and how he will train his new employee.

Most people go through a number of attendants before they find one compatible with their needs. Careful attention to detail during the hiring process helps to avoid many common pitfalls. Advertising announcements should state the specific nature of the job so as not to attract overqualified applicants—nurses, for example, who may refuse after employment to perform non-nursing tasks. During interviews, a full description of expected duties will help weed out poorly qualified or uncertain candidates. All applicants should be screened as to future plans; one who views the job as a stopgap measure might be less desirable than someone with no other employment goals. A frank discussion about wages and other forms of compensation, rules of conduct for live-in help and arrangements for weekend, holiday and sick leave will prevent problems that often develop after employment. Reliability and honesty must be scrupulously checked by personal references. Finally, the establishment of a probationary period allows time for training and assessment before the attendant and employer make a firm commitment.

Medicaid reimburses patients for part-time personal attendants in some states. Other possible financial resources for attendant care include insurance reimbursement from workers' compensation or some other appropriate policy; vocational rehabilitation for persons with vocational goals; Social Security disability benefits; and the Veterans Administration. Furthermore, the cost of an attendant is a tax-deductible medical expense.

HOUSING

Housing is closely related to the issue of personal care since many individuals can be independent only if they live in a barrier-free environment. Most types of home modification are easier to accomplish when a disabled person lives in his own home or rents from an agreeable landlord. Funding sources for modification projects include the Department of Housing and Urban Development (through city and county social service offices); vocational rehabilitation for disabled housewives with family responsibilities; and the Veterans Administration.

The plight of city apartment dwellers is more distressing, because few can afford to live in apartments with elevators, and landlords tend to be uncooperative. Then, too, problems of personal safety detract from the convenience of street-level apartments. Some communities now offer safe and convenient subsidized housing to elderly and disabled people; in addition, 5 percent of all family units in new public housing must now be designed for use by the disabled. Although waiting lists for these units can be long, it still pays to check on them with public housing agencies or offices for the elderly and disabled.

Other housing possibilities include "independent living centers" or other cooperative living arrangements which provide a barrier-free environment and shared services. During the last decade, about 100 independent living centers were established in the United States; plans to develop other centers are now being delayed by funding problems. Hospital rehabilitation social workers can usually be consulted about independent living facilities in their state.

Foster homes and halfway houses are other alternatives for moderately disabled people who cannot modify their own living area and have no family close by. These permit a person to live in a homelike environment where he has companionship, supervision and ready access to his community. Social workers or public health nurses can provide information about local resources that are operated or supervised by public or private agencies. In addition, private arrangements for foster home care are possible when a suitable family can be found; clergy and social workers can often help with this search.

Finally, some mobile-home manufacturers market homes that can be easily modified to accommodate disability. This possibility is best explored with local manufacturers or sales representatives.

TRANSPORTATION AND ARCHITECTURAL ACCESS

Transportation is a critical barrier for many disabled people who want to lead normal lives, because it is the key that unlocks doors to employment, education, recreation and community services. Difficulties with transportation are frequently compounded by difficulties in the use of buildings and public facilities. City and country dwellers have equal trouble with transportation and access. None of these problems have easy solutions.

The Rehabilitation Act of 1973 established federal regulations to improve transportation and architectural access for the disabled. Under its Section 502 guidelines, all new or substantially remodelled buildings and transportation services that receive federal funds are to be constructed to permit full use by disabled people. The Architectural and Transportation Compliance Board was established to receive complaints and enforce the provisions of this act. Although comforting in the abstract, these regulations have proved ineffective because they apply only to projects that receive federal funds, which now more than ever are in short supply. Worse yet, at present federal administrators show a distinct lack of enthusiasm for these regulations, and expend little effort or money to enforce compliance.

Where they exist, comparable state and local laws have more impact, because they regulate a wide variety of building and transportation services including, in some instances, privately financed ones. Enforcement is normally easier to accomplish at a state or local level.

First we will focus on individual solutions to transportation and building access problems. (It should be noted that group effort is far more effective than individual action.)

Many disabled people have no means of transportation whatsoever. They cannot drive or in some cases fit into a car, they have no friends or relatives to help them, their communities lack accessible public transportation and taxis or other private forms of transportation are too costly. When we can provide transportation for our disabled relative, whether for occasional errands or daily trips to work, we do him an invaluable service. But many lack the time or resources to offer, this help.

Reliance on friends for transportation can strain relationships, especially if they are asked to help on a regular basis and suffer great inconvenience or financial loss. To ensure a friend's continuing goodwill and cooperation, we ought to offer some form of payment whenever possible. Sometimes co-workers, fellow students or members of organizations to which a disabled person belongs are willing to provide daily transportation if they are reimbursed for their time and extra costs. Finally, we might try to hire someone with a vehicle and spare time to help out. Newspapers and bulletin boards are good places to advertise for senior citizens, housewives and students who are anxious for additional income. When hiring strangers, we should check personal references, vehicle insurance and driving records.

Many disabled people drive their own vehicles with the aid of adaptive equipment. Vehicle and equipment costs, rather than degree of disability, are often the most limiting factors. Sources for financial assistance include the Veterans Administration, vocational rehabilitation, and private insurance companies. Negotiations with an insurance company for a low-cost or interest-free loan have a better chance of success when it can be shown that a vehicle will permit a person to work and thereby reduce his dependency on disability benefits. In addition, events sponsored by co-workers or service organizations (dinners, dances or raffles, for example) have been used to raise money for people who need specialized vehicles. (Although many disabled people spurn acts of charity, a project that focusses on the needs of a specific individual gives friends and acquaintances a meaningful outlet for their genuine concern.) *The Handicapped Driver's Mobility Guide,* published by the American Automobile Association, supplies excellent information about driving regulations, adaptive devices and vehicles, specialized driving schools and funding sources.

Buses and subways transport large numbers of disabled people, but a general lack of accommodation to many disabilities—the need for a wheelchair, for example—still excludes many who need these services. The cost of adapting public transportation to serve the handicapped population is not prohibitive, but such projects receive low priority when cities are hard pressed for funds. However, changing municipal priorities is not something that individuals can accomplish on their own.

Where specialized door-to-door transportation for the handicapped exists, the cost is often prohibitive—to the point where many people who might otherwise be willing to work are discouraged from doing so. In communities that offer publicly subsidized or voluntary transportation services for the elderly, it is sometimes possible for a disabled person to arrange to use these services even though he does not qualify as elderly.

Most people are familiar with the obvious architectural barriers—stairs, narrow doorways and curbs, for example, that defy negotiation in a wheelchair. Lately handicapped parking signs have been erected, elevators and ramps installed, lavatory stalls widened, and braille characters embedded next to directional signs, and we think that all the problems of architectural access have been solved.

We think so, that is, until we try to help a disabled person keep an appointment or run an errand, suddenly to discover all sorts of barriers that had previously eluded our notice. Even when the disability is minor, we find that doors are too heavy to open or impossible to maneuver through with crutches or a walker. If we are trying to help someone who uses a wheelchair, we find all the handicapped parking spaces occupied by cars of able-bodied people. Business establishments, churches and public buildings that we had previously visited without a second thought are suddenly off limits to our disabled relative. Very quickly we begin to learn more than we ever wanted to know about back entrances and freight elevators.

Despite all the progress in recent years, much still needs to be done to improve architectural access for disabled people. However, when we act as individuals, our complaints about lack of access will be ignored by city officials and business people dragging their able-bodied feet. As individuals trying to help one specific person, our only recourse is to work around these obstacles.

Before our relative ventures out into the community then, we may have to scout out routes, checking for doorways, ramps and elevators, perhaps. If lavatory and eating facilities are inaccessible, we will have to plan accordingly. These preparations are apt to take a great deal of time, especially when a person is severely disabled. But the time and effort we spend paving the way for our relative to return to the community is worthwhile. He may be dismayed by all the difficulties of trying to resume a normal life, but he will be inspired by our determination to make sure that nothing stands in his way.

EMPLOYMENT AND EDUCATION

By far the most serious barriers to employment are unseen. They include the attitudes of the disabled person himself: "Why should I work and lose my disability benefits?" "The world owes me a living because I'm disabled," "I'm worthless and no one will hire me because I don't have any skills," "I'm not going to even try for a job because I can't stand to be turned down."

They are also the attitudes of his family: "We're so busy taking care of him that we don't have time to help him find a job," "Why should he work when it's easier to keep him at home?" "If he worked, he'd lose his disability benefits and we'd be worse off than we are now," "Besides, no one will hire him because he can't even take care of himself."

They are the attitudes of employers: "Sure I feel sorry for disabled people, but I've got my business to run," "If I hire someone with a handicap, my insurance rates will go up," "I don't have time to restructure a job, and I certainly don't have the money to change the facilities in my plant or office!" "My other employees would feel uncomfortable working with someome who is handicapped; it would ruin company morale," "Well, perhaps I can find some simple job for one or two of them. After all, I want to do my bit for those poor folks."

However, the facts about employment of the disabled contradict these attitudes. To address the doubts of the disabled themselves: Often work does provide adequate monetary compensation, but, more significant, it makes a person feel independent, worthwhile and fulfilled. It provides social interaction with others, status in the family and community, and makes leisure time more satisfying. Efforts to promote employment almost always lead to greater emotional and financial rewards for everyone in the family—and those results are well worth any effort.

The fact is that handicapped individuals are good workers. A study by Du Pont found that the handicapped workers in its program had excellent or above-average records in performance, attendance, safety and all other critical areas related to productive employment. All their physically handicapped workers—whether craftsmen, professional managers, technicians, machine operators or service personnel—were as good employment risks as their able-bodied co-workers. Du Pont also found that adjustments in the work area were minimal and acceptance of handicapped workers by other employees was wholehearted.[1]

The experiences of other companies, large and small, concur with the Du Pont findings. Furthermore, Anthony Magliozzi, manager of rehabilitation for the Liberty Mutual Insurance Co., the largest casualty insurer in this country, refutes the contention that workers' compensation rates will go up.

> There is absolutely no way that a company's insurance premiums will rise because it hires disabled individuals. If a company's insurance premiums are experience-rated, rates may rise when employees have accidents, but not because the company has hired someone with a handicap. Higher insurance rates are a myth—a cop-out for employers who are looking for an excuse not to hire a disabled person.[2]

"Hire the handicapped—it makes good business" was a slogan that helped large numbers of handicapped people find work in the fifties and sixties. Unfortunately, now and in the past, most disabled people hold jobs beneath their skills when compared to their able-bodied counterparts with similar education and training. A great majority of these people end up in the "secondary labor force" as seasonal or part-time employees who earn minimum wages and have no benefits or job security.[3] This situation can change only when more employers stop thinking "hire the handicapped" and start hiring qualified people who happen to have handicaps.

Many disabled individuals who want to work have marketable skills; others need education or technical training to prepare them for the work force. Before examining educational opportunities for the latter, we will look at ways to help someone with job skills find suitable employment.

To begin, it is necessary to understand the laws governing employment of disabled people. As with the regulations for architectural access and transportation, federal laws have limited effectiveness because they cover only employers who receive federal funds. State and local statutes are more comprehensive since they regulate a wider variety of employment situations. However, a review of federal laws will suggest some of the opportunities that all these laws are supposed to provide.

Several sections and later amendments of the Rehabilitation Act of 1973 affect the employment and education of the handicapped. Section 501 forbids discrimination against current and prospective employees of the federal government solely on grounds of disability. Section 503 requires non-discrimination and affirmative action by federal contractors and subcontractors on behalf of disabled applicants and employees. Section 504, by far the most comprehensive, states that "no otherwise qualified handicapped individual shall, solely by reason of his handicap, be excluded from participation in, be denied the benefits of, or be subjected to discrimination under any program or activity receiving federal financial assistance." This section affects state and local governments, grade and high schools, colleges and hospitals—anyone with a hand in the federal purse. In addition, the Vietnam Era Veterans' Readjustment Assistance Act of 1972 mandates special provisions—similar to those in Sections 503 and 504 of the Rehabilitation Act—for disabled or economically disadvantaged Vietnam veterans.

To fully appreciate the significance of these federal regulations and their state and local counterparts, we need to understand some commonly used terms:

- *Affirmative action* requires employers to have an equal-treatment program that covers all employment practices, including hiring, recruitment advertising, upgrading, demotion, layoffs, termination, employer-sponsored activities such as social and recreation programs, and any other condition or privilege of employment.
- *Discrimination* refers to any activity that denies services or employment or segregates an individual because of his handicap.
- A *handicapped individual* is any person with a physical or mental impairment that substantially limits one or more major life activities. Handicapping conditions include, but are not limited to, cancer, cerebral palsy, diabetes, epilepsy, heart disease, deafness, blindness, multiple sclerosis, muscular dystrophy and drug or alcohol addiction.
- *Substantially limits* refers to a handicap causing difficulties in securing work or retraining or advancement in employment.
- *Major life activities* involve any activity that has to do with communication, ambulation, self-care, so-

cialization, education, transportation or employ-
ment.
- *Qualified* is a key word that means the individual must be capable of performing the essential tasks of a job, given reasonable accommodation by the employer to his handicapping condition if needed.
- *Reasonable accommodation* refers to making necessary adaptations to enable a qualified handicapped person to work.

Arno Zimmer, in his book *Employing the Handicapped: A Practical Compliance Manual,*[4] gives examples of reasonable accommodation:

- making parking, lavatory, and cafeteria facilities accessible to and usable by handicapped persons
- restructuring jobs to accommodate special needs or modifying work schedules to accommodate transportation difficulties
- equipping a telephone for use by a worker with impaired hearing
- providing readers or interpreters or a cassette recorder for a blind employee
- teaching sign language to the supervisor of a deaf employee
- relocating jobs or offices to accessible buildings
- providing an accessible and adequate workplace for someone with a wheelchair
- allowing time off for a worker to receive treatment at a methadone or alcohol treatment center

By law, employers (and schools) cannot require applicants to furnish information about a handicapping condition. However, an applicant can choose to supply such information if he wants an employer to comply with affirmative action or reasonable accommodation. Medical information is confidential and can be used only to prepare for possible medical emergencies. Although employers are forbidden to automatically screen out disabled applicants, they can deny employment to someone whose disability prevents the performance of necessary job-related tasks—but only when that condition is not amenable to reasonable accommodation. For example, an employer can deny a truck driving job to someone who cannot hold a driver's license because of a handicap.

Under some regulations, screening for disability can be done only after an employee has been hired. If a condition is then found that would prevent him from performing his job, the employer has the right to terminate. Tests and examinations of any sort can be given only to determine those skills and abilities directly related to the job. Reasonable accommodation must be made in testing applicants with an impaired function not specifically related to the job. For example, oral examinations must be available to a blind person or a quadriplegic who cannot write out the answers, if either is otherwise qualified to fill a job.

In summary then, many federal, state and local laws mandate that certain employers provide fair treatment to all people regardless of their handicaps. They must evaluate each person on the basis of his abilities and qualifications for a particular job, rather than on his disabilities. When an applicant qualifies for a job, these employers must accommodate the employee's special needs.

All these regulations have opened up many new jobs to disabled people with marketable skills. Although employer compliance is still poor in some areas, new opportunities are created every day. Our relative stands a better chance of finding a job if we can help him locate potential job openings in companies or institutions that are required to provide equal opportunity to the disabled. To identify such employers, we can suggest that he contact vocational rehabilitation and job service offices or employment agencies with listings of "equal opportunity" employers. Other resources include classified advertisements and friends with special knowledge about job openings.

Before applying for any job, an applicant ought to learn as much as he can about the prospective employer and the job specifications. He will have more success if he identifies a job that suits his abilities and can be adjusted to his disabilities.

Applying for a job is the same for everyone in that it is essentially a process of selling oneself to an employer. The sales pitch is particularly important when the applicant is disabled. He should be optimistic and enthusiastic, and avoid references to his handicap or pleas for sympathy. He should dress neatly and appropriately, and appear for the interview on time and alone. He must stress the value of his abilities, pointing out ways in which he can fill a position to the benefit of his employer. Finally, he should be prepared to suggest how the employer can accommodate his special needs.

Many employers are frightened by the cost of "reasonable accommodation" according to government guidelines. Remodelling the work environment to accommodate an employee who uses a wheelchair, for example, can involve considerable expense. Many times, however, an applicant can suggest simple modifications that are adequate to his needs. He will score extra points with an employer if he suggests possible sources of funding to cover training and accommodation costs. One such source, Target Job Tax Credit, established by the federal Revenue Act of 1978, offers tax credits to employers who hire vocational rehabilitation referrals and economically disadvantaged Vietnam veterans. The Tax Reform Act of 1976 used to permit employers to deduct up to $25,000 from their federal taxes for expenses involved in removing architectural barriers. That act expired in 1982, but some states still allow similar deductions. Job service and vocational rehabilitation counsellors can supply details about Target Job Tax Credits and may have information about state tax credits. Otherwise, one should contact a state tax office.

Some employers have made a voluntary commitment to hire disabled people because they realize the wisdom of such action. Others—even ones legally obliged to do so—are still recalcitrant. If a disabled person is refused employment for a job he is qualified to perform, he can file a complaint. Complaints about federal employers, employers with federal contracts or employers receiving federal funds should be addressed to the appropriate federal regulatory agency.* Complaints regarding employers covered by state or local laws should be directed to the state or municipal agency that deals with employment rights of the handicapped. Vocational rehabilitation counsellors have information about these agencies.

Discrimination complaints, especially those addressed to federal agencies, almost never produce speedy or gratifying results. In fact, there are no records of any federal contracts withdrawn or financial support denied for failure to comply with handicapped employment

---

* For complaints regarding federal employment discrimination: Office of Secretariat, Interagency Commission on Handicapped Employment, Civil Service Commission, 1900 E Street, N.W., Washington, D.C. 20415.

For complaints regarding employers with federal contracts or subcontracts: Office of Federal Contract Compliance Program, Employment Standards Administration, U.S. Department of Labor, 600 D Street, S.W., Washington, D.C. 20201.

For complaints regarding employers receiving federal funds or complaints from applicants who are Vietnam veterans: Office of Civil Rights, Office of the Secretary, U.S. Department of Health & Human Services, 300 Independence Ave., S.W., Washington, D.C. 20201.

regulations. In some instances, however, when an employer has a long history of discrimination, federal agencies have managed to enforce compliance through negotiations. Better results are sometimes obtained at the state or local level.

Although written complaints never produce quick action from government compliance agencies, they often encourage an employer to reconsider and reverse his decision. Filing a complaint is a good idea, then, if the applicant wants to add to a company's history of noncompliance or induce an employer to change his mind. Since most agencies have time limits for filing complaints, it is best to file soon after an incident of suspected discrimination. The applicant should include the following information in his report:

- his own name, address and telephone number
- the name and address of the discriminating company or institution, along with the name of a contact person in that organization
- the nature of his handicap
- the nature of the discriminatory act
- background information relating to the complaint
- copies of relevant correspondence
- his signature

Accurate records of correspondence and other written documents are important evidence for proving discrimination. Employers often deny employment without giving reasons; in order to substantiate a discrimination charge, the job applicant should request that the employer furnish his reasons for denying employment in writing. If necessary, the applicant might send a registered letter asking for this information. An employer's failure to comply with such a request can be used as additional evidence.*

Finding a job is difficult in the best circumstances. When a person is disabled, the inability to obtain work reinforces feelings of inadequacy and uselessness. Typically, most people give up their job search after a few unsuccessful attempts. For our disabled relative to succeed, we must force him to look further and remind him that with his skills he has a *right* to work.

Two alternatives for people with disabilities are self-employment or working at home for an employer. Any type of business venture is possible if a person has the necessary skills. The Small Business

* Legal action to deal with employer discrimination is discussed at the conclusion of this chapter, under "Advocacy: Legal and Group Action."

Administration offers loans, technical assistance (including market analysis to determine the need for a service or goods) and other information to help start a business.* Other resources for starting a business include vocational rehabilitation and the Veterans Administration.

Countless job opportunities exist for people who want to work at home; some that can produce a good income are the following:

- a telephone answering service for companies or professional offices
- a clearinghouse for such services as transportation, rentals of all sorts, housecleaners, babysitters, temporary housekeepers, food caterers or handymen
- duplicating, addressing, typing or printing service for companies, organizations or students
- a writing service to produce letters, brochures, family histories, speeches or grant applications
- a newspaper clipping service for legislators, organizations or companies
- accounting or billing services
- photo developing or picture framing
- tutoring or instruction in music, foreign languages or handicrafts
- plant growing or pet breeding
- ironing, sewing or baking
- a repair service for locks and keys, knives and scissors, small appliances or toys
- production of such items as original crafts or sports clothing from kits

Another newly emerging home occupation involves computers. Several major companies are now hiring disabled individuals to work with computers in their homes.[†]

Traditionally, disabled people working in their homes had to resort to the production of craft items that were boring to make and

* Contact a local SBA office or write to Small Business Administration, 1441 L Street, N.W., Washington, D.C. 20005.
[†] Readers seeking information about companies offering this type of employment in their area should contact local vocational rehabilitation counsellors for information about nearby firms. Another source of information is the director of the HOMEWORK project at Control Data Corporation; write to Public Affairs, HQS13M, Control Data Corporation, P.O. Box O, Minneapolis, Minn. 55440.

almost impossible to sell. Exciting opportunities for home employment exist, however, when individual skills are matched with community needs. Classified ads are a good place to begin this search, but we need not stop there. We can contact companies or organizations to see if they have any jobs that could be filled by someone working at home. For example, a university student might need a typing service, a professional office might be able to use a telephone answering or accounting service or a local store might be willing to sell a homemade product because there is demand for it.

Vocational rehabilitation and Small Business Administration counsellors often can help with this type of community-needs assessment as well as technical assistance and the purchase of necessary equipment. Unfortunately, some vocational rehabilitation counsellors tend to focus only on traditional, boring and poorly paying forms of home work. We may need to stretch imaginations—our own and others'—a bit to come up with an idea that engages our disabled relative's interest and challenges his abilities.

Many communities have strict zoning laws governing the operation of businesses in residential neighborhoods. Authorities sometimes permit a variance in the zoning code if a business is unobtrusive and does not generate additional traffic or parking problems. For services that involve food, local health department regulations should be checked.

Let us turn now from employment—finding work for a disabled person with skills—to education—finding ways to help him acquire the skills he needs to get a job.

Two resources, training programs and "sheltered workshops," offer simultaneous employment and training. CETA (Comprehensive Employment and Training Act) has been replaced by the Job Training Partnership Act, but the new act continues the goals and services of CETA programs—to improve job skills of the unemployed and underemployed. Clients receive classroom training to enhance work skills, subsidized on-the-job training with employers who would not otherwise hire them, or short-term work assignments with businesses. Satisfactory completion of a program often ensures permanent employment with cooperating employers.

Sheltered workshops or "opportunity development centers," as they are sometimes called, are operated by private organizations such as Goodwill Industries or by publicly financed agencies. Some offer long-term employment to individuals who are unable to compete in the regular work force because they may work too slowly or have problems with social adjustment. Other workshops provide job-skill evaluation, on-the-job training and preparation for entry into the labor market. Vocational rehabilitation is the best place to go for information about these services.

Many people involved in rehabilitation think that educational services for the handicapped frequently put too much emphasis on remedial training for the handicap and not enough on job-skill training. For example, blind people need not only to be taught braille but to be trained as teachers, lawyers and mechanics. Concern about education is twofold, then; the disabled person must be trained both to manage with his disability and, depending upon his age, condition and goals, to acquire job skills.

Vocational rehabilitation is a good source of help in assessing an individual's potential in the job market and his educational needs, especially if he has no specific vocational goal in mind. Even if he does know what kind of training he wants, we may need to help him find a source for that training, whether it is a correspondence course, a mini-course at a vocational school or an advanced course of study at a university. Guidance counsellors in high schools, vocational schools, colleges and universities can supply information about courses at their own institutions, as well as resources for home-study, independent-study and tutorial programs. Most libraries have in their reference collections several directories with information about institutions of higher learning, including their programs and facilities for the handicapped. Educational funding resources include vocational rehabilitation, workers' compensation, the Veterans Administration and a variety of financial-aid and work-study programs available through student admissions offices.

Educational institutions that receive federal funds—most of them do—are required to observe the same equal-opportunity regulations as employers. For example, they cannot on the basis of a handicap deny application to anyone otherwise qualified for admittance into a program. They must provide reasonable accommodation in administering admissions tests to applicants with impairments. And they are required by law to provide reasonable accommodation so that handicapped students have full access to buildings, classes, services and school activities. Complaints about suspected discrimination should be directed to school administrators, governing boards, or, ultimately, the Office of Civil Rights in Washington, D.C. Written complaints should include the same information as cases of suspected employment discrimination.*

* See footnote, p. 101 above.

Leisure time can be a curse to the disabled person who has too few interests and no friends. His problems are magnified when he lacks money or access to community activities. If our disabled relative suffers in this way, we can begin to fill the void by suggesting projects that will develop new interests or channel his abilities into enjoyable pastimes. Our suggestions can range from simple arts-and-crafts projects to volunteer work to something as extravagant as a C.B. or ham-operated radio if sufficient money is available.

Although we may be able to provide him with materials or equipment for his use, we will have a far more difficult time supplying him with friends. A disabled person is apt to lose his friends, perhaps because he is no longer good company or cannot participate in previously shared activities. Often, too, he refuses to see old friends because they are an uncomfortable reminder of his former life and thus of his present limitations. His social contacts are further diminished when he lacks opportunities to make new friends or refuses to associate with other disabled people, whom he views as inferior.

We ought to encourage our relative to keep active with his old friends even if his involvement in their activities must be at a new, different level. And we can help him meet new friends by finding people who share interests—for example, fellow stamp collectors, card players or music aficionados. The shame that he feels in associating with other disabled people is likely to disappear when he discovers that many of them are as much fun and have as much to offer as their able-bodied counterparts. Even though he may be very resistant, we should try to involve him in self-help groups where he can meet other disabled people and make new friends.

Free or inexpensive recreational opportunities abound in almost every community. Some people find these services through adult day-care facilities or nursing homes that encourage nonresident participation in weekly card games, parties or dances. The American Red Cross conducts swimming programs for disabled people, and service organizations sponsor parties and programs for them. Other groups offer the disabled free tuition for courses and passes to athletic and concert events. In some localities, able-bodied volunteers have organized to participate with disabled people in such activities as camping, bicycling, skiing, mountain climbing and skydiving. Our eighty-year-old grandmother may not be thrilled by all these ideas, but we should be able to find a few that suit her needs and interests.

Travel requires money, of course. Even those of the disabled with ample financial resources often stay home because they are afraid of encountering insurmountable difficulties if they try to leave their community. Although problems with transportation and access still exist, the news about travel for the handicapped is more encouraging every day. Some airlines, Amtrak, interstate buses and some automobile rental companies now provide special services to the handicapped. Several motel chains offer rooms and services to accommodate disability. Directories list accessible highway rest areas, facilities in national parks, camping sites and access guides to cities in the United States and foreign countries. Several organizations provide travel information, and privately operated travel groups arrange or conduct tours to all parts of the world.

The key to successful travel, especially for disabled people, is advance preparation and careful planning of every detail of the trip. Nothing should be taken for granted. For example, Amtrak now has accessible coaches and lavatory and dining facilities on each train, but some of the railroad stations themselves are still inaccessible to many disabled people. Then, too, definitions of "accessible" vary. Motels with wheelchair-accessible rooms often have bathroom doorways too narrow to accommodate some types of wheelchair. And although airlines almost always have wheelchairs for handicapped passengers, they may not provide attendants to push them.

When making reservations, then, we must ask very specific questions: "Does the airline [or airport or motel] permit guide dogs?" "Does the airline place any restrictions on handicapped passengers?" "What are the charges for handicapped transport services between airport terminals, and how does one arrange for this service?" "Do buildings on the tour have ramps? How wide are the doorways?" "Can arrangements be made for a special diet or emergency medical services?"

Although time-consuming, such careful attention to detail will help to avoid many difficulties associated with travel. The disabled person who has the money to travel should not have to put up with unnecessary frustration and disappointment on his vacation or business trip. He, like the rest of us, deserves a bon voyage.

ADVOCACY: LEGAL AND GROUP ACTION

Supportive attitudes and persistent efforts can do much to restore a disabled person to a normal life in his community. Often these efforts will fail, however, because of barriers that are impervious to individual assault—barriers that can only be overcome by legal action or group effort.

Disabled people are usually in a poor position to be assertive. They often hold themselves in such low esteem that they have neither the conviction nor the courage to demand fair treatment. In trying to cope with the disappointment of disability, they cannot tolerate other disappointments. Consumed with their own day-to-day problems, they do not identify with others who have different disabilities but face similar problems, and seldom join forces with them. They are poorly informed about their rights, and lack both the resources and the will to fight.

For all these reasons, we family members are the ones who must fight their battle against discrimination. We must become informed and demand the enforcement of laws that guarantee equal opportunity. We can hire lawyers to help with legal skirmishes or join self-help or advocacy groups. Where we have failed as individuals, we can succeed by working with others. In the final analysis, legal and political clout may be the only effective weapons in this war.

The case for political action is most graphically demonstrated by recent federal actions regarding Social Security benefits. Threats to diminish Social Security retirement benefits were met with strong resistance by our elderly population, whose organizations brought pressure to bear on federal administrators and legislators. Yet, almost without public notice, new regulations have stripped many deserving people of their Social Security disability benefits. In an effort to conserve Social Security funds, our federal government has picked on those with the least political influence. Further cutbacks in food stamps, job training, medical assistance and many other programs have caused more serious problems for those segments of the disabled population that are poor, unskilled and powerless.

Kenneth Kolpan—director of the Handicapped Education Law Program at Tufts New England Medical Center (until that program became a casualty of federal cutbacks), and now in private law practice in Boston—believes that the major barriers facing disabled people are society's attitudinal problems, all couched in legal terms. In his experience, the administrative complaint process—in which a person files a complaint with an administrative agency on his own behalf—is generally ineffective. He is convinced that legal action through the courts is the only feasible solution for discrimination issues.[5]

We may be unwilling to start legal action if we are uncertain about our disabled relative's legal rights or concerned about legal fees. However, we ought not to decide against this alternative, without more information about available help.

First of all, a number of organizations in this country are working to ensure the rights of the disabled. Some of them, like the American Civil Liberties Union, prefer to become involved only in issues that affect large groups of people; however, others provide assistance to individuals. Social workers in hospital rehabilitation departments are usually familiar with advocacy agencies and legal information clearinghouses in their own state. Some communities have legal-aid services—fewer now because of funding problems—that offer assistance to people with low incomes; lawyers associated with these programs are often knowledgeable about the rights of disabled citizens. In other localities, vocational rehabilitation operates "client assistance" projects to provide legal assistance to disabled individuals.

Lawyers in private practice are another resource for legal counselling. State and local organizations for the handicapped and local bar associations have listings of attorneys who are qualified in the area of disability law. To be sure, private legal services are expensive; however, courts sometimes award attorney fees to successful plaintiffs in cases involving federal regulations, and frequently include reimbursement for legal fees in other types of legal settlements.

Most lawyers will grant a free preliminary interview to discuss a case, but it is best to ask about charges before making an appointment, especially if money is a concern. Legal services are usually based on either an hourly rate or a contingency fee that is a percentage of an award if the case succeeds. With contingency compensation, the lawyer receives no fee if his client loses the case. Sometimes the plaintiff can reduce legal costs by finding others with similar problems and hiring an attorney to handle a group action. Self-help groups have been particularly effective in this regard.

Court action need not always be the end result of consulting an attorney. Lawyers can also provide information about federal, state and local disability laws, appropriate enforcement agencies to contact for discrimination complaints or methods of appeal. (Charges for these services would depend upon the individual lawyer and the time required to obtain the information requested.) Or, we can obtain a lawyer's help in investigating, for example, a pattern of discrimination practiced by an employer. Many aggrieved job applicants and employees have found that merely involving a lawyer in their case convinces an employer to reconsider and negotiate a satisfactory settlement.

Some self-help groups supply a great deal of legal assistance and support. They invite attorneys to their meetings or share their own experiences in trying to gain fair treatment. They spearhead projects involving other community organizations in order to influence government action. Working with high school business classes, for example, they might conduct surveys to determine the architectural accessibility of local business establishments. They often form coalitions with other groups to improve local transportation services for disabled people, work with local chambers of commerce to publish community access guides, and sponsor meetings with business and industrial leaders to encourage employment of the handicapped.

When all else fails, some groups resort to civil disobedience, holding protest demonstrations when municipal services are inaccessible and boycotting businesses that refuse to provide adequate facilities for the handicapped. Slowly, ever so slowly, they are making their voices heard. As they continue to organize and involve more people, both disabled and able-bodied, they will become an important political force in this country.

Someday these groups may succeed in destroying the attitudinal and environmental barriers that prevent disabled people from leading normal lives in the real world. Without doubt, their chances for success would be far greater if all of us with disabled friends and relatives joined them in their efforts.

CHAPTER 7

"How Can We Pay for All This?"

FIRST, THE BAD NEWS: Costs for medical care are doubling every five years. Daily charges for a hospital bed in the early 1960s averaged thirty dollars; today they are between two and five hundred. Now the good news: Many people today recover from conditions that formerly caused death or permanent disability. New surgical procedures replace damaged heart arteries, organs and joints. New devices perform kidney functions, regulate heartbeats and control insulin dosages. New drugs and other treatments successfully treat some cancers and many other diseases.

Although grateful for these advances in medicine, we find their costs staggering, especially if we lack adequate insurance coverage or lose our source of regular income. Then we are bound to ask how we can pay for all this.

The very poor in this country usually qualify for government assistance in paying for medical services and some living expenses; the very wealthy have no real problems because they have enough insurance or other resources to guarantee good care and continuing income. The majority in the middle are less fortunate. Many with moderate income lack adequate insurance, because they either cannot afford to purchase enough coverage, have chosen not to plan for the possibility of serious illness, or have simply lost their insurance along with their jobs during the current recession.

The disabled homemaker is a particular and unexpected financial burden for a family with average income. She is seldom eligible for assistance from government disability programs, and most families do not bother to purchase homemaker disability insurance protection. Her husband's health insurance may cover her hospital bills, but not the costs of hiring someone to care for her personal needs and do her housework. Often she refuses rehabilitation because treatment costs will further deplete the family savings.

Money of course plays a critical role in rehabilitation choices. Although acute or emergency care is usually given regardless of a patient's financial circumstances, this is not the case for rehabilitative treatment. When a patient decides to delay rehabilitation until money is available, his rehabilitation is seriously threatened. Unfortunately, some patients wilfully postpone rehabilitation in order to prove disability and increase the sum of money they hope to receive from disability compensation or a legal settlement.

Disability compensation is justified in many situations—for example, while the patient is undergoing treatment, or when he has no potential for rehabilitation or self-supporting employment. For the majority of disabled people who can respond to treatment, however, the opportunity for permanent disability benefits poses a dangerous threat to recovery because it offers income without work. To collect compensation, a person must prove his inability to work or carry out normal activities; he may even be encouraged by his family or legal advisors to exaggerate the disability so as to collect larger benefits. However, in the process of convincing others that his condition is hopeless, he comes to believe so himself. These benefits may appear attractive because they provide income without work, but the lack of productivity and purpose in life leads to a loss of self-esteem. Rehabilitation does have financial rewards, but these are secondary to the emotional rewards of feeling useful.

We are concerned about money, then, because we want to encourage prompt rehabilitative treatment and ensure that the family will have sufficient income when treatment is long-term or expensive or recovery is impossible. Dr. Don A. Olson, director of the Education and Training Department, the Rehabilitation Institute of Chicago, sums up the problems we face:

How can we better serve the physically disabled in our nation? The shocking fact is that resources are available in most situations, but due to lack of *cooperation, communication* and *consideration* of the needs of the physically disabled, programs falter and the "system" goes against the individuals it was designed to serve.[1]

In the sections that follow, we will look at these resources and some ways to ensure that our disabled relative has every possible advantage. These resources include

- benefits from private health, accident, liability and disability insurance policies
- federal and state programs, including Social Security, Medicare, Medicaid, Supplemental Security Income, Vocational Rehabilitation and Workers' Compensation
- other federal programs that serve special groups
- state and local services administered by social service and public health departments
- local services by private voluntary agencies and organizations

Our disabled relative will not be eligible for all these resources, but there is a good chance he will qualify for more of them than expected. For example, many families with extraordinary medical bills are eligible for Medicaid even when they do not qualify for income assistance programs. Also, many life insurance policies and mortgages and other debt contracts carry clauses that waive payment by the patient in the event of total disability. Insurance or banking agents can advise if such contractual clauses exist and are applicable. In addition, we ought to check for other health, life or disability insurance policies our relative might have purchased in connection with an organization membership or a special occasion such as a trip. In searching for resources, then, we do better to look too far rather than not far enough.

We must be willing to persevere until we find what the patient needs. When we encounter inconsiderate personnel or a tangle of regulations, we must be polite but assertive. And if he is denied a legitimate claim to benefits, we can appeal that decision through a process that is available for all insurance and public assistance programs.

Finally, we ought to keep records of relevant conversations and correspondence to help in tracking down resources, and of medical expenses which will be helpful when the time comes to file claims and income tax reports. Suggestions for record keeping conclude this chapter.

PRIVATE RESOURCES

Health Insurance

Over twelve hundred insurance companies sell medical insurance in this country.[2] As one might expect, the quality of their policies varies greatly. In fact, many people only discover how poor their coverage is when they become sick and use their policies for the first time.

There are five basic types of health insurance: *Hospital expense insurance* pays specific benefits for daily hospital room and board and the "usual hospital services and supplies," up to specified maximum limits. *Surgical expense insurance* pays for surgical procedures, either a certain amount for each type of procedure or the "usual and customary fee" for surgery. *Physician (or medical) expense insurance* pays physician fees for non-surgical care in the hospital, home or doctor's office, sometimes including diagnostic and laboratory charges. All three types of policies have maximum limits on the benefits they pay. Individually, none of them offers adequate coverage for a catastrophic illness requiring lengthy hospitalization and many surgical or medical treatments. A combination of these policies would, however, provide excellent coverage.

Major-medical expense insurance provides broad protection for large, unpredictable medical expenses. It covers a wide range of charges with high maximum benefits and few specific limits. This type of policy usually has a "front-end" or initial expense deductible and then pays 80 percent of eligible expenses. Some comprehensive plans provide both basic and extended coverage; that is, they pay for hospital, surgical and medical charges as well as skilled care provided by a nursing home or home health-care visitors. *Health maintenance organizations* (HMOs) provide comprehensive care to enrolled members in return for a fixed periodic payment. Under such a plan a group of physicians and other health professionals furnishes care in the doctor's office, hospital, nursing home or patient's home. Recently, in an effort to keep their premiums competitive with other types of insurance programs, some HMO plans have begun to require a small initial deductible to discourage overutilization of services and facilities.

114

In addition to the above five basic insurance programs, private supplemental policies are available to people enrolled in the Medicare program. These policies pay for some of the medical expenses not covered by Medicare.

Some Cautions About Health Insurance. Three types of health insurance, although heavily advertised, are not recommended by consumer groups or reputable insurance agents:

Hospital indemnity insurance pays specific sums of money for each day spent in the hospital. The premiums for this type of policy are often excessive, considering that the average hospital stay is less than eight days.

Specific-disease insurance protects the subscriber who falls victim to a particular disease, most commonly cancer or heart disease. The elderly, who especially fear these illnesses, are a target for companies selling this type of insurance. Besides charging excessive premiums for the protection they offer, these policies tend to give their holders a false sense of security. Too often people with such insurance think they have adequate protection. However, they do not consider the wide range of other illnesses that can befall them. Those with a comprehensive medical insurance policy or Medicare and a supplemental policy have no need for this type of insurance.

The elderly, often fearful of being a burden to their families, also fall prey to the purveyors of *nursing-home insurance.* These policies like most other insurance policies, only cover skilled care—not the custodial care most nursing-home residents receive. Nursing-home insurance is thus an unnecessary and expensive duplication for anyone already having Medicare and a good supplemental policy.

Few of us take the time to check our policies until we become sick. In view of today's rapidly rising medical costs, we should give them a periodic evaluation. Some state insurance commissioners supply guidelines for insurance purchase and evaluate insurance companies operating in their jurisdiction. However, it is best to deal with a local agent who can study individual needs, prevent duplication of policy coverage and recommend respected insurance carriers.

Laws in some states allow a person to convert his health insurance from a group to an individual policy if he stops working. These provisions are particularly helpful to a disabled person because he can continue to participate in his group plan even when he is forced to leave work. He must pay the full premiums himself, but group rates are much less than individual rates. A few states also operate high-risk pools for people who were formerly considered medically uninsurable.[3] Local insurance agents are familiar with pools that operate in their state.

One final caution deserves emphasis: *Health insurance companies cancel policies when premiums are not paid promptly.* In the event of disability, the family should make every effort to continue premium payments; otherwise they will lose their medical coverage and be in a poor position to purchase insurance elsewhere.

Filing Health Insurance Claims. Claims for medical expenses are processed either directly through the provider of services (for example, the doctor or hospital) or by reimbursement to the patient after he has paid his bill. Under either system, the insurance company notifies the patient what charges it will pay and what he must pay.

Discrepancies between expected and actual coverage can often be traced to fine print in a policy. When we think a company should be paying more of the expenses, we should write immediately to its customer service department asking for justification of its payment decision. If the company's response is unsatisfactory, we can submit all pertinent information about the claim to the state insurance commissioner. Although not legally binding, his opinion often influences insurance company action.

Automobile and Liability Insurance

Both automobile and liability insurance policies pay medical benefits for injuries sustained in an accident, but many difficulties are associated with their reimbursement policies. Often people with the most serious injuries are the least likely to collect their expenses. They may have to postpone treatment for years until their case is settled. We need to understand these reimbursement systems so we can negotiate to assure prompt medical treatment and reimbursement.

Medical Coverage From Automobile Insurance. Most automobile insurance policies—or those for other vehicles—pay medical expenses for the insured, other family members in the same household or other occupants in his car, regardless of who is at fault in the accident. Family members are also covered under most standard policies for injuries that involve *any* vehicle—whether they are a driver or occupant of another car or a pedestrian.

Reimbursement limits for medical costs are usually one or two thousand dollars per person for each accident; some are higher but rarely exceed five thousand dollars. Most policies set a time limit on reimbursement following an accident for "expenses incurred within one year"; some now extend that to three years.[4] These payments are for "reasonable and necessary" medical costs not covered by any other insurance policy owned by the accident victim; they include charges for medicine and drugs; ambulance and other medical transportation services; nursing, medical and dental care; and medical equipment, eyeglasses and prostheses.

Arranging for Prepayment. The standard time limit phrase, "for expenses incurred within one year," is often questioned, especially in serious accident cases. In general, the courts have allowed an injured person to collect for medical expenses beyond one year—*if* his expenses do not exceed the monetary limits of his policy, and *if* arrangements are made to prepay for anticipated services.[5] This means that a person who expects his treatment to extend beyond one year should pay in advance for those services (up to the amount he is eligible to collect from his policy) and ask his insurance company for an immediate reimbursement. In a few cases the courts have allowed people to collect for services contracted before the expiration date but paid only upon completion of treatment; prepayment is much safer, however.

Regardless of the circumstances of a vehicular accident, we ought to consult our insurance agent immediately for information about benefits. If prolonged treatment is necessary, we should discuss prepayment so as to conform with policy time limits. Doctors and other health professionals should outline a treatment program with cost estimates if they know we are operating under time constraints for reimbursement.

Liability Insurance. People injured through someone else's negligence can file a claim for medical costs, lost wages and other related expenses against the person at fault and his insurance company. Injury may have occurred while in a vehicle, on the premises of a home or business, through negligent service or use of a faulty product, among other causes. Particularly in cases of serious injury, the injured person must prove that someone or some company was negligent and is therefore responsible for his injury.

In liability cases, claim payments are based on either "contributory" or "comparative" negligence. Which category applies depends on the state where the injury occurs. In states with contributory negligence laws, the injured person may not be able to collect payment if he is in any way responsible for his injury. In states with comparative negligence laws, a claimant can collect partial payment depending upon the degree to which he is not at fault for his injury.[6] When a person is judged, for example, to be 30 percent negligent himself, he may still be able to collect up to 70 percent of his expenses.

Recovery of medical expenses from another person's automobile insurance company in a liability case is often difficult, if not impossible. A 1970 report by the U.S. Department of Transportation found that 45 percent of those who are seriously injured in traffic accidents get absolutely nothing from liability insurance.[7] Conditions remain the same today. Those who suffer the least are most likely to collect, often more than their costs; the more serious the injury, the longer until settlement. These statistics are alarming, because the accident victims who most need medical services are denied immediate reimbursement and may in fact never recover their costs from those at fault. (Our concern here is only with medical costs, not, for example, with reimbursement for lost earnings, permanent disfigurement or suffering; these losses involve other inequities in serious injury cases.)

No-Fault Insurance. Approximately twenty-five states now have "no-fault" automobile insurance laws.[8] These laws are supposed to eliminate the need for costly and lengthy litigation to decide liability and claims settlements. In no-fault insurance all injured occupants in a vehicle are entitled to benefits under the policy that covers that vehicle. Injured pedestrians are covered either by their own no-fault policy or by the policy of the driver who caused the injury, depending upon the state.[9]

Payments from no-fault policies to the injured person partially reimburse him for medical expenses, lost earnings and some essential services. The allowable amounts vary with the policy and state law. Whether the no-fault system succeeds is controversial; it seems to work best when injuries are minor or only moderately debilitating, because payment is automatic, immediate and fairly comprehensive. When injuries are more serious, reimbursement limits in some states prevent adequate coverage of medical costs and other expenses. Although the injured person can sometimes sue the negligent driver for additional compensation, the problems of litigation are then the same as in states without no-fault legislation.

Whatever the system, the policyholder's automobile insurance agent should be contacted immediately after an accident to learn how best to proceed with a claim. When serious injury has occurred and someone else is at fault for the accident, an agent can often help negotiate for prompt rehabilitation care.

Advance Payment Settlements in Liability Cases. Advance payments can sometimes be negotiated in cases of serious injury. In such a settlement, the insurance company of the person at fault agrees to advance money for medical expenses (and sometimes lost wages). In order to receive these payments, the injured person is not required to sign any type of release that would waive further claims against the company. Any money advanced to him is then deducted from the final settlement, whenever that occurs.

Some, although far too few, companies have begun to use this form of settlement. They find that advance payments help establish better rapport between the injured person and themselves; also, since the payments ensure prompt treatment they may lessen the final claim. Though it may cost thousands of dollars to rehabilitate a paraplegic, it costs hundreds of thousands to maintain him in custodial care for life.

Companies are often unwilling to make advance payments in accident cases where details of the accident are confused and liability is difficult to establish. However, many states now encourage advance payments, holding that such payments are not an admission of liability.[10]

In the event of an accident, it is best to deal honestly and realistically with claims adjusters. Rather than try for a generous legal settlement some years in the future, we should be concerned only with getting the money needed for immediate rehabilitation. Insurance companies try to avoid the high costs of litigation, and when we convince them that we do not intend to press for excessive compensation if the injured person is able to obtain proper medical care, we improve our chances for getting advance payments.

In 1971, Secretary of Transportation John A. Volpe reported to Congress and the President as follows:

> Three different investigations by the department have demonstrated that despite commendable efforts by the insurance industry to introduce "advance" or partial payment techniques, the system is still, in the main, quite slow in cases where the need for timely payment would appear to be greatest, i.e., in cases of permanent impairment or disfigurement.[11]

Little has changed in the years since that statement. However, the possibility of failure should not deter us from trying. Independent insurance adjuster Roy E. Holloway encourages his fellow adjusters and insurance companies to use advance payments more often:

> The job of the adjuster is to act as a liaison between the rehabilitation professional and the company. He can learn from the professionals what is needed and he can assist in providing those needs through his company.
>
> The sooner the rehab professional can work with a patient, the easier it will be to promote satisfactory results. If the disability victim is delayed in being referred into a rehabilitation process, he is deprived of an opportunity to become active and self-supporting and has, in fact, been given an unneeded opportunity to become depressed, to lose motivation, to become lethargic and to face prolonged economic problems resulting from reduced income. The insurer has lost the opportunity to put rehabilitation dollars to work while paying out, quite probably, much more money in disability payments over an extended period of time.[12]

Not all adjusters are as enlightened as Mr. Holloway. If we cannot obtain advance payments from an insurance company, we may want the advice of an attorney. However, we ought to be suspicious of any lawyer who encourages delay in rehabilitation or exaggeration of disability in order to obtain a larger settlement. In fact, we may have to shop around for one willing to accept the goal of prompt payment for immediate medical services.

Attorneys are generally not needed to settle liability claims under five thousand dollars, because insurance companies tend to pay "small" claims promptly to avoid the cost and inconvenience of litigation. Although an attorney might help to secure a larger settlement, his fees can consume a large portion of the award. However, no matter what the size of the claim, we ought to seek legal advice if we are asked to sign a release form absolving the insurance company from further claims, in negotiating for a prepayment or advance payment settlement.

Structured or Periodic Payments. "Structured" or "periodic" payment settlements are sometimes used in personal injury cases where an individual is severely disabled for life, as with a brain or spinal-cord injury, and damages are expected to exceed one million dollars. Normally in cases of this magnitude the injured person eventually receives his full award in one lump sum. However, in structured payment settlements, the liability insurance company purchases an annuity policy from a life insurance company which makes regular payments to the injured person for his care and support for a period of time, usually until death.

These settlements have advantages and disadvantages.[13] If the injured person dies within a few years, his heirs receive nothing unless specific terms in the agreement provide for a lump sum settlement or continuing support payments to dependents in the event of early death. On the other hand, these payments could amount to substantially more than a lump sum settlement if the individual lives for a long time.

An advantage of large lump-sum cash settlements is that they can yield handsome benefits when invested wisely, although many who receive generous awards fail to get adequate financial advice. However, unlike lump sum settlements, periodic payments have the advantage of avoiding federal and, in most instances, state income taxes. In addition, periodic-payment agreements can be written to accommodate such variables as inflation.

Structured payments are attractive to many patients and their families also because they are often easier to obtain than lump sum settlements. Although they take time to negotiate, there is usually less delay and likelihood of losing a lawsuit. They are appealing to the liability insurance company because it saves money. The premiums paid out by the company for annuity insurance are considerably less than the sum required for an outright cash settlement—even if the injured person eventually receives more than he would from a lump sum settlement.

An attorney with experience in such settlements is essential because the negotiable terms are extremely complex. Legal fees are high, of course, but a skilled attorney can extract his fees from the settlement, independent of the monthly payments awarded to the patient.[14]

Subrogation Clauses. A subrogation clause is commonly written into insurance policies. Briefly, this clause gives an insurance company the legal right to recover from a third party payments it has already made to the policyholder. For example, in the event of an accident, a person's health and automobile insurance companies may have the right to recover money they have previously paid him for medical expenses, from his liability settlement.

This clause is one more reason why litigation should be approached with caution. A patient considering legal action should bear in mind that even if he receives a large settlement, much of his award money will be reclaimed by other insurance companies that have previously paid his medical expenses. Combined with legal fees (up to 50 percent of the settlement) and taxes, these sums greatly deplete his net award.

In the absence of a subrogation clause, the policyholder may be able to collect twice for the same medical expense, perhaps from his own insurance company and a liability carrier or from both his automobile and health insurance policies. Although such instances are rare, we should ask our insurance agent or claims representative about this possibility.[15]

To sum up, when someone is injured in an accident, it may be necessary to negotiate prepayments and advance payments from automobile or liability insurance companies in order to ensure timely rehabilitation—especially if his health insurance policy does not provide sufficient funds. We do him great harm when we encourage legal alternatives that, though they could ultimately provide compensation, nevertheless delay his treatment. Court settlements are almost always financially disappointing, but their greatest disadvantage is the serious emotional consequences of postponed rehabilitation.

FEDERAL PROGRAMS FOR THE DISABLED

The federal government operates or contributes to several programs that pay medical and income-maintenance benefits to the disabled. These include Social Security, Medicare, Medicaid and Supplemental Security Income and state vocational rehabilitation and workers' compensation programs as well as services to other special groups such as veterans.

Although these programs all provide important help, many critics feel they do not properly serve our disabled population. One of them is disability rights advocate Frank Bowe, who says in his *Handicapping America: Barriers to Disabled People,*

> The vast majority of federal funds spent on programs serving disabled people goes not to helping them help themselves through training and job placement, but to income maintenance programs that actually discourage disabled people from seeking work.[16]

Economist William Johnson has severe criticisms of public disability programs. Although his comments reflect data collected by the Social Security Administration in 1972, they are equally applicable to the SSA's most recently published figures. He notes that one-half of the men and nearly three-quarters of the women who are severely disabled receive no benefits, often because their disability was not the result of employment or military service. Many people fail to receive benefits because they are unaware of their eligibility. On the other hand some disabled people receive benefits from two or more programs because of serious duplication problems.[17]

Even among those in our disabled population who currently receive government assistance, a significant proportion lack sufficient income to pay for their most basic needs; those who are most disabled are the poorest. For example, latest SSA figures show that one-fourth of the severely disabled fall below government poverty guidelines, despite the fact that slightly more than half of them receive assistance.[18]

In 1981, the Social Security Administration paid $17.3 billion in disability benefits to 4.5 million disabled workers and their dependents; the Supplemental Security Income program dispersed $5.7 billion to 2.3 million low-income people who are disabled or blind. Despite these astounding sums of money, many social workers, lawyers, psychiatrists and consumer groups are critical of a 1980 law that requires a stringent review of disability cases. They charge that many eligible—and desperately needy—disabled people have lost their benefits through arbitrary and overzealous enforcement of this law. People with mental ailments have been particularly vulnerable to federal cutbacks. Although they constitute only 11 percent of the disabled population, one-third of their number have been removed from disability roles, leaving them without income or job prospects.[19]

People fall through the cracks in the government system because they are either unaware of their eligibility or unqualified for programs under current federal guidelines. Disabled homemakers are particularly vulnerable in this last regard. And some disabled people and their families are too proud to ask for help; they refuse to accept public assistance even though their taxes have supported these insurance programs for many years.

Despite their many problems, government programs can still be a valuable resource. Constantly changing guidelines and funding levels and state variations in administration and benefits make detailed description of each program impossible. Nevertheless, a review of their services and application procedures will suggest many avenues to explore.

Social Security Administration

Disability Benefits. The Social Security Administration provides benefits to disabled workers and their dependents through several programs, one being the disability benefits program. To be eligible for these benefits, a worker must have been covered by Social Security insurance long enough to have accumulated sufficient work credits; this time requirement varies with the age of the worker. Disability benefits are available to all eligible workers under the age of sixty-five. (Those over sixty-five are covered by Social Security retirement benefits.) Dependents may be entitled to payments if an insured parent or spouse receives Social Security retirement or disability benefits or is deceased. For example, some spouses of deceased Social Security beneficiaries may qualify for benefits if they become disabled after the age of fifty.

All these benefits are part of the Social Security insurance program, which is funded by worker and employer contributions. They are designed to replace some of the potential earnings lost due to disability or death. The size of the monthly payment is based on the worker's average earnings while he was contributing to the program; it is not based on need—at least at the time of this writing. Anyone who is enrolled in Social Security, applies and is judged disabled automatically receives benefits, regardless of income.

The Social Security Administration considers an individual disabled when he cannot work for his income because of a severe mental or physical condition. For dependents, the inability either to work or to carry out normal, daily living activities constitutes disability. The condition need not be permanent, but it must be expected to last at least one year or result in death. Upon application, payments start with the sixth full month of disability and continue for the duration of the condition.

Workers who become disabled from a work-related accident or disease can receive both workers' compensation and Social Security disability benefits, but limits are placed on the amount of the combined benefits. These limitations do not affect payments a worker might receive from a private disability insurance program.

Medicare Benefits. The Social Security Administration's Medicare health insurance program assists the elderly or severely disabled to pay their medical expenses. This program has two aspects: hospital insurance and medical insurance.

Anyone who receives Social Security disability benefits for twenty-four months is automatically enrolled in the Medicare hospital insurance program. Benefits include hospitalization, skilled nursing-home care and home health visits. Payments are made for "reasonable costs" of necessary drugs, supplies, appliances and other equipment and services given to patients in a hospital or skilled nursing facility. Home health services include part-time skilled nursing care; physical, occupational and speech therapy; medical social services; and medical supplies and equipment provided by a home health agency. There are deductibles and limitations on the amounts paid under this program.

Medicare medical insurance can be purchased for a small fee, which, if the recipient chooses, can be automatically deducted from his monthly disability benefit. This program pays for physician and hospital out-patient care and certain other medical items and services not covered by Medicare hospital insurance. Here again, there are deductibles and limitations on benefits.

People with Medicare hospital and medical insurance can also purchase a Medicare supplemental insurance policy from a private company. These policies pay for some of the costs not covered by the two Medicare programs. Since the quality of these supplemental policies varies greatly, it is best to deal with a trusted local agent who can evaluate family needs.

It should be noted that workers enrolled in the Social Security program who have permanent kidney failure and need maintenance dialysis or a kidney transplant are eligible for Medicare benefits, as are their dependents.

Supplemental Security Income. The Social Security Administration directs the Supplemental Security Income (SSI) program for people of any age who are blind or disabled. Unlike Social Security disability benefits, eligibility and the amount of SSI payments are based exclusively on financial need. (Persons who receive Social Security disability benefits invariably have too much income to qualify for SSI.) Any blind or disabled person (even someone who has never been enrolled in the Social Security insurance program) is eligible for SSI benefits if he has little or no regular cash income and very few assets that can be turned into cash. Property of very modest value—such as perhaps a house, car, household and personal effects or insurance policies—is often exempted when considering eligibility. No claims are placed against real or personal property holdings when a person is enrolled in SSI.

To qualify as disabled under SSI guidelines, a person must be unable to work because of a mental or physical condition that is expected to last at least a year or result in death. To be classified as blind, he must be unable to read with corrective lenses below the top line on an eye chart or have a severely restricted field of vision.

Each state sets its own guidelines for eligibility for and amount of SSI benefits; rarely do these payments provide more than a bare minimum for living expenses. All but eight states (Arkansas, Kansas, Louisiana, Mississippi, Ohio, Tennessee, Texas and West Virginia) add a supplement to their residents' SSI payments. Some states conduct additional needs evaluations and issue separate monthly checks; others automatically include their allocations in the checks sent by the federal government.

SSI recipients normally qualify for Medicaid—which pays for necessary medical expenses—without any waiting period.*

Work Regulations for Social Security Programs. In the past, many disabled Social Security recipients who had an opportunity to work did not do so, because they would have automatically lost their monthly payment and Medicare or Medicaid protection. (Sometimes these benefits have exceeded potential after-tax earnings from work if an individual required costly medical care.) Changes in Social Security work regulations now encourage disabled individuals to return to work.

People who have not fully recovered from disability are entitled to a trial work period of up to one year, during which disability payments continue. Medicare coverage continues for three years after the worker starts earning a substantial income, but only if he has not made a complete recovery. SSI and Medicaid recipients can continue to receive benefits after they return to work, even if their earnings exceed normal income limits, but payments decrease as earnings increase.

Most encouraging of all, certain expenses—such as medical care and equipment, attendant care and support services necessary for daily living (for example, specialized transportation)—can be deducted from the worker's income figure in calculating his ability to earn a living wage. For example, one person who must spend a large share of income to pay an attendant might still qualify for benefits,

---

* Since Medicaid is administered at the county level, application procedures are explained later in this chapter under the heading, "Public Social Service Agencies."

while another earning the same amount but with few disability expenses might not.

These very laudable changes help disabled people who are able and eager to earn a living. They do not always help people who, though they cannot be self-sufficient, still can earn part of their living expenses. Understandably, many of these people refuse to sacrifice the financial security of their benefits for the emotional and psychological advantages of working and feeling productive.

Application for Social Security Benefits. We should not hesitate to call a Social Security office if there is *any* chance for benefits; there are no foolish questions when Social Security monthly payments are at stake. These offices are listed in the white pages of the telephone directory. Calls placed after the middle of the month are more likely to receive prompt attention. Counsellors can start an application over the telephone and specify what additional information they need to complete the claim. Anyone applying for Social Security benefits has a right to question decisions about his claim or the amount of his benefits. Social Security personnel will assist with this appeals process.

Veterans Administration Benefits

Veterans Administration programs provide medical care, disability compensation and other special services to veterans and their dependents. Any veteran, or anyone closely related to a disabled or deceased veteran, may qualify for assistance.

Medical Care. Although any veteran may be eligible for medical care in a VA hospital or skilled nursing-care facility, preference is given to those with disabilities resulting from military service; other veterans are served when beds and funds are available. Certain veterans also qualify for out-patient treatment at VA facilities, out-patient dental care, prosthetic appliances, other aids, services to the blind and deaf and treatment for drug and alcohol dependence. Rehabilitation services to eligible veterans include an annual clothing allowance to compensate for unusual wear caused by a prosthesis or wheelchair, assistance in purchasing an automobile or other special conveyance, and reimbursement for adaptive equipment needed to operate a motor vehicle.

Disability Compensation. Veterans disabled by an injury or disease incurred during active service, or aggravated by it, can receive disability compensation. In fact, veterans who develop a disease after their service may be eligible for benefits if they can demonstrate that their condition is directly related to military service. Disabilities associated with nuclear testing during World War II, the psychological trauma of service in Vietnam and exposure to Agent Orange now receive considerable, but not undisputatious, attention. Such conditions as tropical disease, leprosy, tuberculosis and multiple sclerosis are presumed to have been caused by military service if they appear within a specific time after discharge. The degree of disability and number of dependents determine the amount of disability compensation.

Wartime veterans with disabilities that are permanent and total but not connected with military service may be eligible for pension benefits if their income is limited. The amount of allowance varies with income, number of dependents, living arrangements and care requirements.

Other VA Benefits for Veterans and Dependents. Veterans' dependents and survivors are entitled to VA medical benefits and financial assistance when they do not qualify for help from other sources. Eligibility requirements, too numerous to detail here, involve the veteran's service record and disability history and the family's financial and treatment needs.

The VA also helps some veterans, and dependents of deceased veterans who are themselves disabled, with home financing, home modification to accommodate disability, rehabilitation, education and job training.*

Application for Veterans Benefits. As mentioned above, eligibility guidelines for veterans' benefits are complicated; one need only remember that any veteran or close relative of a disabled or deceased veteran may qualify for help. Toll-free numbers for VA offices are usually listed in the telephone directory under the heading "U.S. Government." VA counsellors will supply forms and specify documents needed to process a claim.

Because VA application forms are difficult to complete, twenty-eight recognized service organizations—including the American Legion, American Red Cross, Disabled Veterans, and Veterans of Foreign Wars—will help any veteran or family with their claim. Contact the local chapter of any veterans' service organization for assistance.

Veterans and dependents can appeal decisions made by the VA

* Programs for disabled veterans who want to return to the work force were described in Chapter 6.

regarding a claim or benefit amount. VA counsellors will provide the necessary forms, but here again service organizations are helpful in preparing an appeal.

Veterans Insurance Programs. Veterans who have GI Life Insurance, Servicemen's Group Life Insurance or Veterans Group Life Insurance may be entitled to disability income benefits, disability premium-payment waivers or monthly payments from the proceeds of their policies. Questions regarding these policies can be directed to VA counsellors or service officers in veterans' organizations.

Federal Programs for Special Groups

The federal government also runs a number of programs for special groups. Civil Service employees hired before 1984, members of the armed forces and railroad workers, for example, are enrolled in special programs with benefits similar to Social Security. Other programs serve such groups as the Merchant Marine, American Indians and migrant workers. Employers or social service counsellors affiliated with these groups can supply information about services and eligibility guidelines.

STATE PROGRAMS

Workers' Compensation and Vocational Rehabilitation

Workers' compensation and vocational rehabilitation primarily serve disabled workers, although a few homemakers are eligible for vocational rehabilitation services. While their administration, funding and services are different, many of their goals are similar. In fact, thirty states have cooperative agreements between their workers' compensation and vocational rehabilitation agencies.[20]

Despite these agreements, many people contend that the two services' procedures are uncooperative, if not antagonistic. These criticisms are relevant here because they show the problems that disabled workers encounter in trying to deal with these agencies. Moreover, they demonstrate once again that many well-intentioned government programs actually discourage rehabilitation. Before reviewing criticisms of these two agencies, let us examine the services they are designed to provide.

Workers' Compensation Benefits. Workers' compensation is state-administered insurance for public and private employees that pays medical and other benefits when an employee incurs a work-related injury or illness. In a few states, workers also receive benefits for disability resulting from non-occupational injury or disease. This program is financed by employer contributions and covers all but a few employees. It distributes four types of benefits: medical expenses, wage replacement, compensation for permanent disability and death benefits.

Through their workers' compensation insurance program, employers are obliged to pay *all* reasonable medical expenses related to on-the-job injury or disease for the duration of treatment. In addition, workers receive wage-replacement benefits to partly replace income lost during the treatment period. This weekly payment, a portion of the average weekly wage prior to disability, varies greatly from state to state. Alaskan workers, for example, can collect benefits eight times higher than Mississippi workers.[21] Depending on his state, a worker must wait from three to seven days before he can begin to collect wage-replacement benefits. Payments continue while the worker is receiving treatment or convalescing for up to twenty-six weeks. If the employee can return to part-time work, even when his recovery is incomplete, he receives partial wage-replacement payments.

At the end of the treatment period, a worker's doctor may decide that he has a permanent disability which is either "total" or "partial." Under workers' compensation guidelines, a person is totally disabled if he has no reasonable chance of earning a living. (However, some seriously disabled workers are classified as totally disabled even though they are not without employment opportunities.) Persons with less severe disability receive partial disability payments. Many states require an assessment of a worker's employment potential as well as his physical condition—considering such personal factors as training, education, prior work experience, job availability and the likelihood of successful rehabilitation—before a determination of disability is made.

Death benefits are paid to dependents of an employee whose death is caused by a work-related accident or disease. The amount of payment is directly related to the worker's former wage, and in some states to the number of dependent minor children. Each state sets maximum allowable limits for death benefits.

Many employees eligible to receive Social Security disability benefits continue to receive workers' compensation disability benefits; however, federal regulations now limit the combined amount a worker can collect from these two programs. Workers' compensation payments for disability or death are not affected by private insurance benefits an employee or his dependents receive.

Application for Workers' Compensation. Workers' compensation claims should be made directly to the employer or the employer's insurance company immediately following an accident or diagnosis of a work-related disease. If the worker thinks he is not receiving all his entitled benefits, he or his family can contact the state workers' compensation board for information about appeal procedure. Counsellors with vocational rehabilitation or job service programs can help with claims and appeal applications.

Vocational Rehabilitation Services. The vocational rehabilitation program was established by Congress in 1921 to return the industrially injured to the work force. Using federal and state funds, this program provides a number of services, including payment for medical care in some instances, to disabled persons who cannot find work. When the program was started, injured workers were the target group. Since the 1940s, Congress has directed that increased emphasis be placed on a succession of other groups—the mentally ill and retarded, handicapped youth, the disadvantaged, those with behavioral problems and disabled Vietnam War veterans.[22] Eligibility for vocational rehabilitation services is based on an individual's desire to work and an expectation that his chances for employment will be improved by these services.

Unlike workers' compensation, which in most states covers only people with work-related injury or disease, anyone with a disability that prevents employment is potentially eligible for vocational rehabilitation services. Many people are referred to these services by their doctor, social worker, employer, insurance company or other health care provider, but anyone can contact a vocational rehabilitation office directly. Each applicant is evaluated to assess the extent of disability and need for services. Any diagnostic work needed to complete this evaluation, including medical examination and psychological and aptitude testing, is paid for by the vocational rehabilitation agency, even if the applicant is ultimately deemed ineligible for services.

States differ in priority assigned to disabled applicants and services provided, but enrolled clients are usually eligible for many services regardless of financial need. These include job placement assistance, counselling to improve job-seeking skills and personal adjustment; tuition and books for enrollment at approved schools;

and skill training in rehabilitation facilities or sheltered work-shops.*

Clients with limited financial resources are also eligible to receive full or partial payment for such services as medical and psychiatric treatment and physical and occupational therapy, and such equipment as prostheses, orthopedic appliances, wheelchairs, eyeglasses and hearing aids.

Vocational rehabilitation also provides special services to the vision- and hearing-impaired to help with adjustment to daily living and preparation for employment. Although disabled homemakers are not eligible for many of those vocational rehabilitation services that relate to the work force, they can receive help with home modification when homemaking is a woman's primary vocation and obstacles in the home prevent her from performing her tasks. Modifications include kitchen and bathroom adaptation, widening doorways, or building ramps to accommodate a wheelchair.

Application for Vocational Rehabilitation Services. Regional offices and local centers for vocational rehabilitation are listed in the white pages of the telephone directory under the state heading. Since applicants must furnish proof of disability (and financial need, when requesting certain medical services), it is best to call ahead to learn what documents are needed for the first interview. Applicants who feel they have been unjustly denied services or are entitled to more benefits can appeal to the state vocational rehabilitation office. Local vocational rehabilitation or job service counsellors will assist with these appeals.

Criticisms of Workers' Compensation and Vocational Rehabilitation Programs. Without question, workers' compensation and vocational rehabilitation help many disabled workers. Unfortunately, aspects of these programs also hurt or neglect many other disabled people who should benefit from their support and services. We will examine criticisms of these agencies here, not to detract from the good that they do, but to learn how to help someone eligible for their services in obtaining what he needs.

To begin, we must face the fact that the availability of generous disability benefits, from workers' compensation or any other source, can seriously threaten a person's desire for rehabilitation. This

* Many of these work-related services were discussed above in Chapter 6.

problem has been well described by George P. Sawyer, a former executive with Liberty Mutual Insurance Company:

> We hear a great deal about the work ethic and how the dignity of work increases self-esteem. The work habit has been a contributing factor in the prosperity of the people in this nation. The primary reason the majority of people work is money. Work for income is a practical alternative to the deprivation of such things as food, clothing and shelter. As such, desire to work has been highlighted as a powerful motivator for people seeking to rehabilitate themselves. As disability income benefits approach the take-home pay of working, a major incentive for a significant proportion of the population is dulled if not lost. Work is probably among the easiest of habits to break if people can gain the things they want without it. When disability is rewarded by sufficient income to satisfy personal wants, making return to work the end product of rehabilitation is seriously threatened.[23]

Although our federal and state governments pay out vast sums to assist people with disabilities, very little of this money is used to encourage rehabilitation—even when people are willing to work for reasons other than financial reward. In *Handicapping America*, Frank Bowe says,

> Rehabilitation, specifically the federal-state vocational rehabilitation program inaugurated by the Rehabilitation Services Administration, has contributed greatly to the alleviation of unemployment and underemployment of disabled people. In fact, congressional oversight hearings consistently demonstrate that for every dollar expended in rehabilitation to disabled people, about nine dollars are returned to the government through taxes by the now-employed or upgraded individuals. Yet in the confusion of priorities, less than 2 percent of every twenty billion dollars spent annually by sixty-one federal programs that serve disabled people is allocated to train them for employment. Most of the money goes to income maintenance.[24]

Sociologist Constantina Safilios-Rothschild has pointed out a number of problems with workers' compensation procedures, noting that disabled workers are not encouraged to receive high-quality medical care. Since income maintenance during rehabilitation is often inadequate to support a worker and his family, he may give up treatment and concentrate on obtaining maximum disability benefits. Lawyers may seriously obstruct rehabilitation by encouraging their clients to seek large cash settlements. Workers are sometimes resistant to attempts to improve their condition because evidence of recovery will reduce their benefits. Finally, Safilios-Rothschild says the self-serving interests of workers' compensation insurance carriers and vocational rehabilitation counsellors cause poor cooperation between agencies and delay the start of effective vocational rehabilitation.[25]

Others have said that insurance companies do not try to encourage disabled workers to reach their full potential through rehabilitation; instead they try to get them to return to any work, no matter how demeaning, so as to reduce disability payments.[26]

Donald E. Falvin, director of Michigan's Division of Vocational Rehabilitation, reports that many vocational rehabilitation counsellors have a difficult time dealing with all the people involved in workers' compensation cases—the insurance carrier, the employer and possibly lawyers—who have no knowledge of the services required to carry out a rehabilitation plan. He says, "It's simply too much trouble for the vocational rehabilitation counsellor to go after the money that is needed."[27]

Many workers who are eligible for workers' compensation fail to apply for benefits because they do not realize their condition is work-related, or they are already covered by other programs.[28] And some employers discourage application for benefits because they are afraid their premiums will rise.

Most states try to enforce prompt payment of disability benefits to workers injured on the job, but a 1980 Department of Labor study has found that the average waiting period for payments to begin is two months. Workers who suffer from work-related disease have a more difficult time collecting benefits. This study notes that about two million people under the age of sixty-five are totally or partially disabled by job-related disease, but only 5 percent of the severely ill get workers' compensation.

The Department of Labor report asserts that many times a job-related disease takes from fifteen to twenty years to develop, and the worker has difficulty proving that the work caused it. Diseases frequently associated with working conditions include emphysema, lung cancer, skin ulcers, circulation problems, heart conditions, permanent back and spine ailments and a variety of lung and blood problems resulting from exposure to irritating or toxic agents. Finally, three-fifths of all disease claims are initially denied, and more than half are eventually settled by a small, lump-sum payment.[29]

States are slow in coming to terms with occupational disease and few cases are reported now. Numbers are expected to rise dramatically during the next ten to twenty years as public awareness increases.

Organized labor sees many reasons why workers' compensation fails to do a good job in rehabilitating injured workers. Lawrence Smedley, an AFL-CIO executive, explains one of them as follows:

Twenty-three state laws deny a worker the free choice of a qualified physician. Few workers suffer severe injury without some psychological overtones; most are pessimistic and depressed. They may feel that they are less than whole human beings. There is a tendency to give up and to think in terms of money needed to make life as bearable as possible for what seems to them an inevitable period of useless obsolescence. Injured workers in this situation need someone they can trust and who can give them good advice, and there is no one in a more stategic position than the physician. However, if the physician is chosen by the employer or insurance carrier, he may not have the trust of the worker. If it is a contested case, the worker is apt to be outright hostile or suspect that rehabilitation advice is an attempt to save the employer and insurance carrier money.[30]

Many physicians as well find fault with both workers' compensation and vocational rehabilitation procedures. They report poor communication in these programs. Patients are frequently sent to doctors for disability or work evaluation without background information about the physical requirement of their employment options. The fact that many patients are as confused as their doctors about the purpose of the examination indicates that counsellors from these agencies often fail to involve their clients in rehabilitation plans.

Finally, many criticize the emphasis vocational rehabilitation counsellors place on retraining for new skills, when injured workers would be better served by finding work that uses their existing labor skills. Eleanor M. Ross, rehabilitation director of the North Carolina Industrial Commission says, "Mature adults who have worked for years in the labor force are very reluctant when one suggests returning to school. Many counsellors seem to feel this reluctance indicates that the client is not interested in vocational rehabilitation services and close the case because of 'non-interest'."[31] As a result, the client is denied access to medical and rehabilitation services.

In summary, workers' compensation pays medical and income benefits to employees with work-related disabilities—almost always for injuries, less frequently for diseases where fault is difficult to establish. Vocational rehabilitation offers services, which may include payment for medical care, to qualifying people with employment potential. However, these agencies often inadvertently encourage many disabled people to seek generous disability benefits instead of rehabilitation.

Our goal should be to ensure prompt rehabilitation and sufficient income during our relative's treatment period; we ought to consider permanent disability benefits only when recovery and employment are impossible.

To tap these two resources most effectively we must first convince the patient that rehabilitation is to his ultimate advantage. Then we must convince his employer and his employer's workers' compensation insurance company that immediate and high-quality rehabilitative treatment for him is to their financial advantage. Finally, we must encourage good communication between insurance adjusters, rehabilitation counsellors and health care providers; they must all work together *with the patient* to devise a rehabilitation plan that serves his immediate and long-term emotional, physical and financial needs.

If we are willing to make the effort to ensure open, honest and constructive communication between all the people involved in our relative's case, chances are very good that we can achieve our goals.

LOCAL COMMUNITY PROGRAMS

Public Social Service Agencies. Contrary to popular opinion, city and county social service ("welfare") agencies offer services that can be used by anyone, regardless of income. For example, they generally have information about many community resources, including the following:

* people who perform homemaking and chore services
* community agencies that help the elderly and disabled
* contractors with experience in home modifications for the disabled
* funding agencies that help disabled people with home modification, including insulation and improvements to sanitary facilities
* agencies and organizations that offer care services

to disabled children and adults so that family members can work or get temporary relief from full-time care responsibilities
- private community organizations that provide emergency funds and other services to the needy
- counsellors who help deal with emotional and family problems

Other social service programs are available only to people with limited income and cash assets or with exceptionally high medical bills. These services include Aid to Families With Dependent Children (AFDC), Supplemental Security Income (SSI), Medicaid, food stamps and the fuel assistance program. AFDC and SSI are financial assistance programs for people with little or no income. The Medicaid program entitles eligible people to free medical and, sometimes, dental care. Food stamps are issued to low-income people to be used as cash for the purchase of food at cooperating grocery stores. The fuel assistance program partially reimburses low-income households for fuel costs. Eligibility for all these programs differs in each state, but often people are eligible for Medicaid, food stamps and fuel assistance even when their income and assets are too high for them to qualify for direct income assistance.

Social service or welfare offices are listed under a city or county heading in the white pages of the telephone directory. Since these agencies usually require proof of income, assets and expenses with any type of financial aid application, it is best to call beforehand. Having necessary information available at the time of application will lessen the waiting period before payments start.

Public-Health Nursing Departments. Public health nurses accept all kinds of calls for help of a medical nature. When not delivered free of charge, costs for these services are based on ability to pay. These nurses are invariably familiar with community groups that offer the free loan of sickroom equipment and free or inexpensive drugs and supplies for certain medical conditions, and with helpful service organizations. They may also have information about medical clinics that treat specific conditions and offer subsidized care to people in financial need.

Private Community Agencies and Organizations. All but the smallest communities have a number of private organizations and agencies that offer help:

- visiting nurse associations or other private home health-care agencies
- religiously affiliated social service agencies or clubs that help the disabled, elderly and needy
- service organizations, such as Lions Clubs that help the blind
- labor unions and veterans' organizations that provide services to disabled members
- local chapters of national organizations that serve people with particular disabilities and diseases, such as the American Cancer Society

Chambers of commerce, United Way offices and crisis intervention "hot lines" (as well as social workers and public health nurses) are good sources of information about these types of local groups.

Public Libraries. Large public libraries frequently offer information and referral service focussing on community resources, but even a small library with no such formal program can be an excellent resource. Library collections usually include many books and periodicals with helpful information for disabled people. One such publication, *Accent on Living* (a quarterly periodical), offers its own information and referral service with extensive files of resources.

Literally hundreds of resources are available to help disabled people. Sometimes these resources are difficult for us to obtain when we encounter inefficient agencies or inconsiderate personnel. Usually, however, the greatest obstacles to finding the right resources are of our own making: pride and the refusal to ask for help, lack of information and unwillingness to learn, and discouragement and the tendency to give up after a few unsuccessful attempts. We *can* find the services needed for successful rehabilitation if we are convinced of ultimate success. And in most cases a little perseverance will carry us a long way.

RECORD KEEPING

Record keeping is a bother, especially considering all the demands placed on our time when a relative becomes disabled, but it can be very helpful in many ways. One of these is in tracking down resources. For that reason, it is a good idea to keep a notebook in which to record important points in conversations with agency and insurance company personnel, including names and telephone numbers. Particularly in dealing with large outfits, this information will expedite future calls or correspondence. In addition, office workers are likely to expend more effort when they realize that the client knows them by name and wants to work with them personally.

A notebook is also useful for recording resource suggestions from social workers, doctors, nurses and other disabled people and their families. Accurate details—names, addresses and telephone numbers of specific individuals to contact—will help to get better and faster service. We should keep copies of all correspondence, in case we have problems with a claim. Accurate financial records are necessary for filing income tax returns, recovering losses from insurance companies or proving financial need. Medical expenses should be tabulated; they are usually tax deductible, and, of course, are needed for insurance claims. In an automobile accident, for example, reimbursement for medical expenses not covered by a health insurance policy can be collected from the automobile insurance policy (up to the limits of that policy) if they can be verified. Copies of bills, payment receipts and cancelled checks can all be used to document medical and related charges for a variety of services and equipment, including the following:

- doctors, dentists and other specialists
- registered and practical nurses; occupational, physical and speech therapists; aides and attendants
- clinic, hospital and nursing home care
- x-rays, laboratory and other diagnostic tests
- medicines, drugs and other pharmaceutical supplies, including dressings and food for special diets
- rental or purchase of wheelchair, crutches, special bed, bedpan, and other sickroom supplies
- prostheses, orthopedic braces, eyeglasses, false teeth, wig for medically caused hair loss, hearing aid and guide dog
- ambulance fees and personal transportation expenses to and from examinations and treatments
- necessary home and vehicle modifications to accommodate disability
- other expenses incurred as the result of disability, such as babysitter, housekeeper, and food and lodging away from home

Documentation of previous earnings is often needed in filing an insurance claim.[32] Salaried persons can collect earnings records from their employers or use past tax records. When commissions or overtime pay formed a substantial part of the income, a letter from an employer is usually enough evidence. Self-employed people can prove previous earnings through appropriate tax records.

Other forms of income, including tips or benefits such as free room and board, can also be tabulated and documented by an employer. "Lost wages" can be established for persons who normally receive no reimbursement for their work—for example, housewives, who can claim lost wages on an insurance claim if they are unable to perform their tasks. A "fair market value" for homemakers is computed by using the local hourly rate for a full-time domestic servant or the national minimum wage. Women with partial disability, who can perform only some household tasks, can adjust these figures for "partial lost wages." Unsalaried workers in a family business or on a family farm can use this method to tabulate their income losses.

Other people who should tabulate lost income for insurance claims include persons forced by disability to take a less profitable job or to work only part-time, or family members who must quit work to care for a disabled relative.

Although most of us are used to opening our financial records to tax people, we are more reluctant to share such private information with an insurance claims adjuster. This is ill-founded, as insurance adjuster Daniel Baldyga says in his book, *How to Settle Your Own Insurance Claim:*

> You shouldn't feel uneasy about letting a stranger peek at your books. In the first place, just remember that the adjuster has to pore over such documents day in and day out with each and every claimant. In the second place, you should remind yourself that if you don't like producing these private and federal documents alone in the privacy of your home, your other alternative (if you want to prove your damages and collect adequate compensation) is to produce them in front of a judge and jury in the wide-open, non-private atmosphere of the courtroom.[33]

Nor should we be reluctant to show strangers our financial records when we want to prove a need for financial assistance. Social workers see far too many applications to remember the details of any; moreover, they are obliged to keep this information in strict confidence.

The U.S. Internal Revenue Service assists with tax reports, as do state revenue services. The IRS distributes two relevant publications, *Tax Information for Handicapped and Disabled Individuals* and *Disability Payments.*

The method used to keep records is not important as long they are accurate, complete and readily available. A daily journal is useful for logging out-of-pocket purchases, mileage and other expenses. Or else pertinent records can be collected in a cardboard box. Bookkeeping chores may seem frivolous, but a simple, convenient system requires little effort to maintain. The actual time spent on this task is negligible compared to that we could waste trying to retrieve misplaced records.

Records, then, help in our search for needed resources and are important in documenting expenses and lost income. If we need financial resources to pay for our relative's rehabilitation, these records will help document his eligibility for benefits.

Medical costs for treatment and rehabilitation are often staggering, but we can meet these expenses if we are determined to find and use every available resource.

Yet, however great the medical costs, the emotional costs of disability are far more disturbing, and require a quite different set of resources. To meet these costs, we must summon from within ourselves every bit of love, patience, understanding, courage and humor we can muster. When we offer these gifts to our disabled relative in large and frequent doses he will learn to adjust to his disability and lead a fulfilling life once more.

Turkeys and Eagles

IN GATHERING INFORMATION FOR THIS BOOK, I met and interviewed dozens of people who are physically disabled. Each of these people displayed some special quality that attracted my admiration and even envy for their accomplishments.

My interview sample is admittedly skewed because I specifically sought out people who are well-adjusted to their disability. I felt I understood the many reasons why some people never adjust to their handicap; I wanted then to find out how and why others were so successful. In every instance, these disabled people reported that family members or close friends had played a critical role in their adjustment.

Some said they would not have recovered emotionally from their disability had it not been for certain family members. Others clearly would have adjusted to their disability in any environment, because they obviously had vast quantities of self-reliance and determination. Yet, even among the latter group, most of them attributed the speed, if not the fact, of their recovery to help from loving people who cared.

Among all the people I interviewed, one individual stands out. Although his adjustment required several years—much longer than any other person with whom I spoke—his testimony strongly, eloquently reinforces the suggestions I offer in this book. I single him out here for special attention because he taught me a lesson about "turkeys" and "eagles."

Charles Sabatier, Jr. is paraplegic. I met him in his Boston office, where he is assistant director of the Massachusetts Office of Handicapped Affairs. I had asked for an appointment after hearing of his recent arrest for disorderly conduct. As I talked to him, pulling my chair close to catch his words, I wondered how and why this soft-spoken, well-dressed executive had come to be arrested.

Charlie—"Please call me Charlie, all my friends do"—doesn't mince words. "I'm today's nigger. I paid my dues in Vietnam. I'm not asking for special treatment; I only want what every able-bodied person has." Getting what able-bodied people have doesn't come easy, Charlie says. Sometimes, on the other hand, he gets singled out for special treatment even when he doesn't want it.

On the day of his arrest, Charlie was boarding an airplane in his wheelchair. He was scheduled to meet with a conference of mayors in Miami to discuss the creation of municipal agencies for handicapped affairs. As he entered the plane, he was told that he would have to sit on a blanket because he was handicapped. When he asked why he needed to have a blanket, the flight attendant told him the blanket would help to evacuate him from the plane in the event of an accident. "But if there's an accident," Charlie replied, "most of the people on the plane will be disabled. Shouldn't everyone sit on a blanket?"

In relating this incident to me, Charlie added, "I had been writing letters to this airline and the FAA for three years, trying to get them to rescind that regulation. They aren't worried about an aircraft accident or my safety; they think that anyone who uses a wheelchair is going to be incontinent and ruin their upholstery. The whole situation reeks of prejudice."

Then other flight attendants became involved in the discussion, and finally one of them told Charlie the plane could not take off unless he used a blanket. Hearing that threat, a passenger screamed at Charlie, "My wife and I have been planning this vacation for twenty years. Don't you dare spoil it for us!"

Unwilling to ruin anyone's vacation plans, Charlie agreed to use a blanket—but only if all the other passengers were supplied with blankets. When several passengers began to chant, "We want blankets, we want blankets!" state patrolmen entered the plane and arrested Charlie for disorderly conduct.

Taken to a police station for booking, Charlie learned he would have to pay a fifteen dollar surcharge to have a clerk called into the station to fill out the forms, because it was a holiday. When he objected to the surcharge, he was told he could either pay it or spend the night in jail. In the end, the second alternative was ruled out and Charlie had to pay the surcharge, because none of the cells or lavatories in the jail could accommodate his wheelchair.

He encountered more accessibility problems the following week at his scheduled court appearance when he found that all the courtrooms were located up flights of stairs and there were no elevators. He refused to crawl or be carried into the courtroom and insisted instead that the judge hold his hearing in the only accessible room in the building—the entrance hall. Charlie told the judge that he would be humiliated by being carried or having to crawl up flights of stairs to plead his case. The judge, however, later complained to reporters that Charlie's behavior had "degraded the dignity of the court."

A few weeks later, Charlie was back before the same judge, but his case had been transferred to a different courthouse, one with an accessible courtroom. By then the airline had reached a settlement with him and his attorney. They agreed to a change of policy, offering blankets to paraplegics only as an option, rather than as a condition of flight. Further, they agreed to pay Charlie twenty-five hundred dollars for attorney's fees and other expenses.

"I won that case, but it was a victory for all handicapped persons," he told me.

"If that airline was so unreasonable, at least at first, why didn't you just fly on an airline that no longer had a blanket policy?" I asked.

"I had planned to fly a different airline until something came up at the last minute and I had to change my ticket," he said. Then, shifting his six-foot, two-inch frame in his wheelchair, Charlie leaned forward on his elbows to make his point. "But this policy was unjust and it *had* to be changed eventually. When this fuss hit the news media, all kinds of people became aware of the problem and they joined in the fight. That's what it takes to change things—a coalition of able-bodied and disabled people working together. It's impossible to do *anything* on your own."

I asked how and where he had learned to be a fighter.

"Disabled people fall into two groups," Charlie said. "There are the turkeys who huddle in little ghettos. They're timid and afraid.

They refuse to take chances, but they're willing to take handouts. Then there are the eagles. They're willing to break away, to take chances on their own. They're the ones who are out soaring, looking for opportunities and willing to fight. It took me seven years to decide that I would rather be an eagle than a turkey."

Charlie joined the ranks of the disabled in Vietnam in 1968. His company was flushing snipers out of a Vietnamese rubber plantation. While answering a wounded friend's screams for help, he was shot through the spine and lungs. Moments later his friend died, but his body shielded Charlie from further bullets. Charlie was finally rescued and airlifted to Saigon. Out of the sixty-eight men in his company, thirty-three died and nineteen others were wounded in that single engagement. In Saigon an enemy attack on his hospital killed eleven nurses. He was eventually transferred to medical facilities in Japan.

"When I enlisted in the Army, they sent me to West Germany, but I couldn't stand all that cold and snow after being raised in Texas. I wanted something warmer and more exciting, so I asked to be transferred." He looked at me and laughed. "*That* was the dumbest thing I ever did in my life!"

"You fought in an unpopular war, you almost lost your life and you became paralyzed. How did you overcome all the pain and bitterness to become the person you are today? Who helped you?" I asked.

"It wasn't easy," he answered. "It took me seven years to adjust, and along the way I went through everything that you read about. I'm a classic case. I've got to give the most credit to my mother. She was the one who really helped me in the beginning."

Charlie's parents divorced when he was fifteen, and he spent a few years living alternately with each parent before going into the service. By the time of his hospitalization in Saigon and Japan, his mother was living in the State of Washington. When he was ready for transfer from Japan to a VA hospital in the U.S., he requested placement in the Tacoma, Washington facility so that he could be near her.

"But when she came to visit me, I was horrible. I'll never forgive myself for the things I said to her. I hated myself and everyone around me. I was constantly testing my family—almost trying to get them to hate me. My mother took it all. She never got angry or seemed personally offended by my behavior. I don't know... Maybe she talked to someone and got some help. She was really terrific."

Charlie's anger spilled out in all directions during the year he spent in Tacoma. He was busted from sergeant to specialist fourth class for speeding down hospital corridors in his wheelchair. He refused to participate in a bowel training program in the hospital because twenty men were expected to use the toilet facilities all together in one room without privacy curtains.

"Sure, I suppose they were afraid we might fall off the stools, and they wanted to catch us, but I wanted to be treated as a person and have a little privacy.

"Much later I had to go into a VA hospital in Texas. There I was, on a stretcher in the hall with no clothes on—just a little drape on my middle. All sorts of visitors were around, but a doctor came up to me and whipped the towel off to examine me right there in front of everyone. He must have thought I was a hunk of meat instead of a person. I wouldn't let that happen to me today, I can tell you!"

Charlie had other reasons for wanting to be in Tacoma, rather than Texas where his roots are. "I didn't want to be near my friends. I didn't think they could tolerate my anger, and I was afraid I'd lose them. Besides, I was ashamed of my body."

Eventually, after a full year in the Tacoma VA hospital, Charlie did return to Texas. He credits his three closest friends with helping him to adjust.

"Good friends know how to behave. They accept you as a person. They seem to have an extra awareness or sensitivity. My disability never seemed to matter to them. They involved me in all their plans. If they were going water-skiing, I drove the boat. They always figured a way so that I could participate—not in the old way, perhaps, but some way. They carried me into some pretty strange places."

"But isn't being carried humiliating?" I asked.

"Being carried is okay when it's my decision," he explained. "If there are two restaurants—one that's accessible with mediocre food and one that's inaccessible with excellent food—I'll be carried into the excellent restaurant. I'm not crazy. But to retain my dignity, I want to make the decision myself."

Along the way, Charlie went to college. "I had to force myself to go out because I was ashamed to be seen in a wheelchair," he said. He also operated a home construction business with some friends. His friendships and social contacts were limited, however, because he didn't want to associate with other disabled people. "I thought they were inferior, and I didn't want my old friends to think I was inferior, too."

Then he ran into a high school buddy who had become paralyzed before Charlie entered the service. "I used to think that if I were like him, I'd kill myself. And there I was, just like him—only he was playing basketball!" After much persuasion, Charlie joined a wheelchair basketball team, only to discover that some of his teammates were far more adept than he, even though more disabled. "At that point I decided I'd better get myself in shape. I lost weight and exercised until I was really fit."

Some time later, after buying a house in Houston, Charlie became president of the local Paralyzed Veterans Association, a group that had given him much support. He helped start a wheelchair repair business which earned thousands of dollars for the association. His interest in veterans' advocacy finally led to a position in Washington, D.C. as national advocacy director for the Paralyzed Veterans Association. He resigned from that position when he decided to help all disabled people rather than just veterans, who often have many government services available to them.

After moving to Massachusetts, Charlie married a young woman who, although legally blind, subsequently graduated from Boston University with a degree in Urban Planning. [Since my interview she has undergone surgery to partially restore her sight.] Both Charlie and his wife are members of the Metropolitan Boston Transit Authority Special Needs Advisory Committee. Charlie is highly critical of an MBTA policy that provides free transportation to the legally blind but does not allow people who use wheelchairs to use their buses.

"They shouldn't be giving free service to anyone until they have sufficient funds to modify their equipment so they can serve everyone. I almost gave my life to this country; I hurt so badly I prayed to die. Now I work, and I pay taxes to subsidize a public transit system I can't get on. I know people who could be earning twenty-five thousand dollars a year, but they can't get to work. They have to stay home and collect disability payments. When that happens, everybody loses!"

Charlie told me, a few weeks after my interview with him, that a group of people were staging a "crawl-in" demonstration in Boston. Since MBTA regulations forbid wheelchairs on buses, paraplegics planned to abandon their chairs and enter the buses by crawling or dragging themselves onto the vehicles. Charlie said, "You have to resort to civil disobedience when authorities are unreasonable. It's the only way to educate the public, to make them aware of what's going on. You have to make fun of the regulations. It's the Boston Tea Party all over again.

"Disabled people are not asking for pity or special attention," he continued. "We're only asking for equal treatment—in this case a chance to use public transportation like everyone else. Too many people have succumbed to the 'telethon' syndrome. Those things are terrible. It used to be that only the handicapped were allowed to beg—remember the blind men who used to sit on corners selling pencils? Well, those telethons are big begging parties. They turn handicapped people into objects of pity. They stigmatize, stereotype and isolate the disabled. People give money to telethons and think that they've done their bit, that they're helping disabled people. Well, they're not."

According to Charlie, "Handicapped people will have to band together and set up their own civil rights movement if they want to improve their lot. Right now, most disabled people don't identify with other disabled people who have a different kind of disability. But even though our needs may be slightly different, we have to work together, because we have a common goal."

Nineteen eighty-one was supposed to be the "Year of the Disabled," but Charlie remembers it as the "Year of Dismantled Programs." "The federal government is now spending even less money on programs to help disabled people. Take enforcement of the Rehabilitation Act of 1973. I have never seen a case where the federal government has withheld funds because a company, agency or organization failed to comply with federal regulations that are supposed to protect the handicapped. Ninety percent of the people who file complaints never follow through. It's just too frustrating trying to deal with the government.

"The trouble is that people in responsible positions are behaving irresponsibly. My legs may be paralyzed, but their *minds* are paralyzed. We can open doors, but we can't open minds."

Since my interview with Charlie in 1982, the federal government's policy regarding the concerns of the disabled has regressed further. For example, less money is available now for modification of public transportation and buildings, and new federal regulations allow more restrictions on air travel by disabled passengers. Old, hard-fought victories are being reversed daily. People in responsible positions are still insensitive to the needs of our disabled population.

Changing the world so that it becomes accessible to everyone is not an impossible task. As individuals we can open doors and clear little paths for our own disabled relatives or friends. But we will never be able to make their world truly accessible until we join forces with others to demand equal opportunity for all disabled people. If we care, we *can* help.

Organizations for Various Disabilities

ALL DISABILITIES

Accent on Living   P.O. Box 726, Bloomington, IL 61701

Operates computerized retrieval system which provides information about resources to help the disabled. (Small service charge waived for those who cannot afford to pay.) Free listing of services and special publications on request. Publishes *Accent on Living,* a quarterly magazine featuring new products, ideas, techniques, places to go, things to do and ways to enjoy life.

AFL-CIO Department of Community Service
815 16th St., Washington, DC 20006 • (202) 637-5189

Serves members of affiliated unions through rehabilitation programs for the mentally and physically handicapped, including counselling for alcohol and drug abuse. Contact a local union representative.

Courage Center
3915 Golden Valley Rd., Golden Valley, MN 55422 • (612)588-0811

Provides rehabilitation and recreational services to people with physical disabilities, including speech, hearing and visual impairments. Offers seventy local and regional programs as well as a transitional residential program at the Center. Free brochure describing services available on request.

Disabled American Veterans
>P.O. Box 14301, Cincinnati, OH 45214 • (606) 441-7300

Offers a variety of services to honorably discharged veterans with service-connected disabilities, and to their dependents and survivors. Special emphasis on Vietnam veterans. Write to national office for information about nearest local outreach office. Publishes *DAV*, a monthly magazine for members.

General Services Administration
>18th and F Streets, N.W., Washington, DC 20405 • (202) 655-4000

Distributes free brochure, *Federal Information Centers*, which lists sources of information about federal programs and agencies to help with specific problems.

National Easter Seal Society
>2023 West Ogden Ave., Chicago, IL 60612 • (312) 243-8400

Provides care through diagnostic clinics and rehabilitation and treatment centers. Programs include sheltered workshops, homebound employment, recreation, provisions for special equipment, social services, psychiatric services, information and referral. Write to Information Office at above address for publication catalog.

National Library Service for the Blind and Physically Handicapped
>Library of Congress, 1291 Taylor St., N.W.,
>Washington, DC 20542 • (202) 287-5100

Provides listening materials for people who cannot read because of physical impairment, as well as information about other resources available to the physically handicapped. Information and application forms are available from local public libraries. (See section below, "Blindness and Visual Impairment," for further services to the blind.)

The National Rehabilitation Information Center
>The Catholic University of America,
>4407 Eighth St., N.E., Washington, DC 20017 • (202) 635-5822

Supplies information from its computerized data base and collection of rehabilitation research reports, audio-visual materials, reference books and journals to anyone who is disabled or works with disabled people. Newsletter, *Pathfinder*, available on request.

Office for Handicapped Individuals
Room 338D, Hubert H. Humphrey Building, 200 Independence Ave., S.W.,
>Washington, DC 20201 • (202) 245-1961

Serves as clearinghouse for information about services to the handicapped. Distributes free brochure, *Pocket Guide to Federal Help for the Disabled Person.*

Rehabilitation Gazette
>4502 Maryland Ave., St. Louis, MO 63108 • (314) 361-0475

Annually publishes *Rehabilitation Gazette*, with current information about education, employment, equipment, recreation and other resources. Discount price for the disabled.

Sister Kenny Institute   Abbott-Northwestern Hospital, 2727 Chicago Ave.,
Minneapolis, MN 55407 • (612) 874-4175

Offers educational materials on adaptation for the disabled: home management, clothing, self-care, movement and lifting, sexual adjustment, bowel and bladder care, care of colostomies and iliostomies, communication problems for stroke patients and nutrition. Catalog and price list available on request.

Social Security Administration   Local or regional office

Operates Medicare, Medicaid, and the disability benefits and Supplemental Security Income programs. Pamphlets include: *If You Become Disabled; Disabled? Find Out About Social Security Disability Benefits; Vocational Rehabilitation for the Blind and Disabled; SSI for the Aged, Blind and Disabled.*

ALCOHOLISM

Al-Anon Family Group Headquarters and Ala-Teen
P.O. Box 182, Madison Square Station, New York, NY 10010 • (212) 475-6110

Sponsors mutual support groups for families and children of alcoholics, and supplies information about local chapters. Write for free brochure, *Al-Anon: Family Treatment in Alcoholism.*

Alcoholics Anonymous World Services
P.O. Box 459, Grand Central Station, New York, NY 10017 • (212) 686-1100

Sponsors local self-help groups for alcoholics and their families. Supplies information about local groups. Write for free brochure, *This Is AA.*

National Clearing House for Alcohol Information
P.O. Box 2345, Rockville, MD 20852 • (301) 468-2600

Offers free literature about alcoholism and treatment services. Send for *Description of Services and Ordering Instructions.*

Women for Sobriety, Inc.
P.O. Box 618, Quakertown, PA 18951 • (215) 536-8026

Sponsors self-help groups for women with drinking problems. Publishes free brochure, *Are You a Woman Who Drinks to Cope?*, information about local groups, and a monthly newsletter.

AMPUTATION

Accent on Living Publications
P.O. Box 700, Bloomington, IL 61701 • (309) 378-2961

Publishes twenty-five page booklet, *Single-Handed: A Book for Persons With the Use of Only One Hand,* which describes devices and products to aid the one-handed person. Covers clothing, grooming, home management, recreation and eating; also contains information about product sources and special interest publications.

National Amputation Foundation
> 12-45 150th St., Whitestone, NY 11357 • (212) 767-0596

This national organization serving amputee veterans operates a prosthetic center for medical and comprehensive rehabilitation services (provides some services to civilian amputees as well); publishes a monthly newsletter, *The AMP;* distributes helpful brochures, including *Pre-Prosthetic Care for Below-Knee Amputees* and *Amputee Guide: Above the Knee.*

ARTHRITIS

Arthritis Foundation
> 3400 Peachtree Rd., Suite 1101, Atlanta, GA 30326 • (404) 266-0795

Operates Arthritis Clinical Research Centers and sponsors local chapters in almost every state. Distributes a number of helpful booklets and leaflets free, as well as the *Self-Help Manual for Patients With Arthritis.*

Arthritis Information Clearinghouse
> P.O. Box 34427, Bethesda, MD 20034 • (301) 881-9411

Catalog of free patient education materials available on request.

Merck, Sharpe and Dohme
> Public Education Department, West Point, PA 19486 • (215) 661-5000

Distributes *Self-Help Devices for Arthritic Patients,* a twenty-page booklet which describes devices for arthritic and other disabled persons.

ASTHMA AND ALLERGIES

Asthma and Allergy Foundation of America
> 19 W. 44th St., New York, NY 10036 • (212) 921-9100

Sponsors local chapters, as well as asthma and allergy hot lines in some parts of the country; distributes publications on asthma and allergic conditions; publishes a quarterly newsletter, *In Touch.*

BLINDNESS AND VISUAL IMPAIRMENT

American Foundation for the Blind
> 15 W. 16th St., New York, NY 10011 • (212) 620-2000

Serves as clearinghouse for information on blindness and services to the blind, including adaptive devices, legal assistance, rehabilitation services, guide dogs and travel. Catalog describes many free or modestly priced publications with excellent information. Aids and appliances catalog offers products for the blind and visually impaired.

Blinded Veterans Association
> 1735 DeSales St.,N.W., Washington, DC 20036 • (202) 347-4010

Serves any blind veteran free of charge. Provides counselling and assistance in obtaining benefits and employment, and promotes advocacy for the blind.

Choice Magazine Listening

P.O. Box 10, Port Washington, NY 11050 • (516) 833-8280

Non-profit organization offers free subscription service to people who are blind, visually impaired or physically handicapped. Bimonthly eight-hour recordings feature diverse variety of magazine articles to be used with Library of Congress playback equipment.

Guide Dogs for the Blind

P.O. Box 1200, San Rafael, CA 94902 • (415) 479-4000

Provides free guide dogs to qualifying blind individuals who desire to increase their mobility and independence. Applicants are usually required to pay their own transportation to the training program. Applicants must be at least sixteen years old, legally blind and have good character references.

Guiding Eyes for the Blind

250 E. Hartsdale Ave., Hartsdale, NY 10530 • (914) 723-2223

Operates a training school in Yorktown Heights, N.Y., which provides guide dogs to qualifying blind individuals. A small fee covers the cost of the dog and training services.

Hadley School for the Blind

700 Elm St., Winnetka, IL 60093 • (312) 446-8111 or (800) 323-4238

Offers free correspondence courses in braille, as well as high school and college courses, to blind and deaf-blind people throughout the world. Courses are provided in braille or on recording. Program information and course catalog on request.

Helen Keller National Center

111 Middle Neck Rd., Sand Point, NY 11050 • (516) 944-8900

Funded by Congress, this organization serves as a resource center for professional workers, and provides comprehensive rehabilitative services to deaf-blind youths and adults. In addition, nine regional representatives offer a wide range of free services.

Independent Living Aids

11 Commercial St., Plainview, NY 11803 • (516) 681-8288

Sells aids and appliances for the blind and visually impaired, including watches, canes, kitchen aids and appliances, recreational and personal aids, and tools and instruments. Free catalog on request.

Leader Dogs for the Blind

1039 S. Rochester Rd., Rochester, MN 48063 • (313) 651-9011

Offers free leader dogs and training to qualified blind individuals from all over the country. Contact a local Lions Club for referral to the training center.

National Association for the Visually Handicapped

305 E. 24th St., New York, NY 10010 • (212) 899-3141

Serves people with partial vision. Prints and distributes large print books; offers counselling and support services, information about optical aids, and referral to local low-vision centers; publishes a newsletter, *Seeing Clearly*. Catalog lists free publications.

National Braille Association
654A Goodwin Ave., Midland Park, NJ 07432 • (201) 447-1484

Operates a braille book bank of professional and educational materials, and provides other transcription services to visually impaired people who have learned to read braille.

National Eye Institute   Building 31, Rm. 6A-32, Bethesda, MD 20205
Office of Scientific Reporting   • (301) 496-5248

Distributes free literature about a variety of eye conditions; publishes monograph, *Low Vision,* describing services available for people with low vision or blindness, including clinics and counselling.

National Federation of the Blind   1800 Johnson St., Baltimore, MD 21230
National Center for the Blind   • (301) 659-9314

National Information Center answers questions about blindness and rights of the blind by phone or mail, offers individual counselling and support services to the newly blind, sponsors local chapters and promotes advocacy for concerns of the blind, publishes a monthly newsletter, *Braille Monitor,* in braille, print and on recordings.

National Library Service for the Blind and Physically Handicapped
Library of Congress, 1291 Taylor St., N.W.,
Washington, DC 20542 • (202) 287-5100

Federal funds provide free services to the blind and those who cannot read because of a temporary or permanent impairment. Services include large-print, braille and recorded books and magazines; playback equipment for recordings; and braille volunteers. Application forms, catalogs or recordings, and catalogs of aids and appliances for the blind and visually and physically handicapped are available from public libraries or regional Library of Congress centers.

National Public Radio Service for the Print Handicapped
2025 M St., N.W., Washington, DC 20036 • (202) 822-2000

Supplies programming to local radio stations that operate reading services for people with visual or reading impairments. Individuals who qualify are given decoding devices from local stations to receive special programming of news, features and entertainment. Contact National Public Radio or state affiliates for information.

National Retinitis Pigmentosa Foundation
8331 Mindale Circle, Baltimore, MD 21207 • (301) 655-1011

Sponsors research into the cause, treatment and prevention of retinitis pigmentosa and other related diseases, provides genetic counselling and referral to treatment centers, sponsors local support chapters and volunteer information centers. Free literature on request.

Recorded Periodicals
>919 Walnut St., 8th floor, Philadelphia, PA 19107 • (215) 627-0600

Publishes scientific and technical periodicals on tape for people with visual impairment.

Recordings for the Blind
>215 E. 58th St., New York, NY 10022 • (212) 751-0860

Supplies taped educational materials to blind and other perceptually and physically handicapped students free of charge.

The Seeing Eye   Morristown, NJ 07960 • (201) 539-4425

Offers guide dogs to qualifying blind individuals from all over the country. A small charge covers all expenses including travel. Free brochure, *If Blindness Occurs,* is available on request.

Social Security Administration   Local or regional office

Provides a variety of benefits and services to people who are blind. Publications include: *Disability Benefits for Blind People; SSI for the Aged and Blind;* and *Vocational Rehabilitation for the Blind and Disabled.*

Telephone companies   Local business offices

Supply information about adaptive equipment to facilitate use of telephones by people with visual impairments.

BOWEL DISEASE

National Foundation for Ileitis and Colitis
>295 Madison Ave., New York, NY 10017 • (212) 685-3440

Serves patients having inflammatory bowel disease, through patient, physician and public education. Local chapters sponsor mutual support groups for patients and their families and offer referral to competent physicians. Distributes literature and publishes a newsletter, *Foundation Focus.*

United Ostomy Association
>2001 W. Beverly Blvd., Los Angeles, CA 90057 • (213) 413-5510

Distributes literature to patients with urinary ostomies, ileostomies and colostomies, and sponsors local chapters for mutual aid and moral support. Publishes *Ostomy Quarterly,* which contains helpful information for patients.

BURNS

The Phoenix Society
>11 Rust Hill Rd., Levittown, PA 19056 • (215) 946-4788

Nationwide self-help organization for burn victims and their families; helps ease psychosocial adjustment of severely burned and disfigured persons during and after hospitalization, sponsors self-help groups, offers counselling by members to burn victims, publishes a quarterly newsletter, *The Icarus File.* Write for free information about nearest area coordinator.

CANCER

American Cancer Society
777 Third Ave., New York, NY 10017 • (212) 371-2900

Offers patient education and services, information about treatment centers, and programs for support and rehabilitation. Some local chapters lend equipment, provide dressings and medicines, help with medical transportation and counsel on finances. Write national or state office to find local support chapters for I Can Cope (for people with cancer), International Association of Laryngectomees, or Reach to Recovery (for women with mastectomies).

Leukemia Society of America
800 Second Ave., New York, NY 10017 • (212) 575-8484

Promotes research and serves patients with leukemia, Hodgkin's disease and lymphomas; distributes free literature about serious blood disorders. Local chapters offer financial assistance for medical care to needy patients and referral to other community agencies. Contact national office for location of nearest chapter.

Make Today Count   P.O. Box 303, Burlington, IA 52601 • (319) 753-6521

Offers peer emotional support through more than two hundred chapters comprising cancer patients and their families, who try to maintain a general goal of living each day as fully and completely as possible. Write to national office for information about nearest local group.

National Cancer Institute   Building 31, Rm. 10A18, Bethesda, MD 20205
Office of Cancer Communications   • (800) 492-6600

Operates Cancer Information Service, a toll-free hot line supplying information about cancer and resources available to cancer patients, including treatment facilities, home care assistance and transportation services; distributes free information about cancer, its causes and treatment, as well as publications about specific types of cancer and guidelines for patients undergoing therapy.

The National Hospice Organization
301 Tower, Suite 506, 301 Maple Ave., W., Vienna, VA 22181 • (804) 243-5900

Provides literature, information and referral to local and regional resources that offer compassionate care to terminally ill cancer patients.

CRANIOFACIAL DEFORMITIES

Society for the Rehabilitation of the Facially Disfigured
550 First Ave., New York, NY 10016 • (212) 679-1534

Aids people with facial disfigurement through clinical services, professional training and public education; provides patient services at NYU Medical

Center; refers out-of-town patients to competent plastic surgeons or plastic surgery clinics in their area.

The Debbie Fox Foundation
P.O. Box 11982, Chattanooga, TN 37401 • (615) 266-1632

Assists persons all over the country who have craniofacial deformities resulting from birth defects or injuries; serves as resource center for information and referral and maintains registry of medical centers specializing in reconstructive surgery; provides support services such as transportation, food and lodging to applicants who qualify based on financial need.

DEAFNESS AND HEARING IMPAIRMENT

Alexander Graham Bell Association for the Deaf
3417 Volta Place, N.W., Washington, DC 20007 • (202) 337-5220

Serves as resource for hearing-impaired children, youths, adults and their families. Distributes pamphlets on many subjects, including hearing aids and lip reading. Free catalog on request.

American Humane Association   1500 W. Tufts Ave., Englewood, CO 80110
Hearing Dog Program   • (303) 762-0342

Provides well-trained free dogs to anyone over the age of twenty-one who is deaf and lives alone or with other hearing-impaired persons. Dogs are trained to respond to such sounds as a telephone, alarm clock, baby crying, burglars, smoke alarm, door knock or door bell. Recipients participate in a five-to-seven-day training program.

Design Center for the Deaf
Dept. of Environmental Design
Rochester Institute of Technology   Rochester, NY 14623 • (716) 464-1653

Publishes a brochure which details modifications to accommodate hearing impairment: *Interior Design Considerations for the Hearing Impaired.*

National Institute of Neurological and Communicative Disorders
Information Office, Bethesda, MD 20014 • (202) 496-4000

Distributes publications, free of charge, including *Hearing Loss* and *Acoustic Neuroma.*

National Association of the Deaf
814 Thayer Ave., Silver Spring, MD 20910 • (301) 587-1788

Promotes the social, educational and economic well-being of deaf people, supplies information about teletypewriting services and other resources that facilitate telephone communication, offers a number of excellent publications dealing with deafness and the problems deaf people face, publishes a monthly magazine, *The Deaf American.* Free catalog on request.

National Information Center on Deafness   T-6, 800 Florida Ave., N.E.,
Gallaudet College   Washington, DC 20002 • (202) 651-5109

Provides information about hearing loss and how to adjust to it within the family and social circle. Gives information on educational opportunities, legal rights, and programs and services for people with hearing problems. Free catalog of publications on request.

Organization for Use of the Telephone
P.O. Box 175, Owings Mills, MD 21117 • (301) 655-1827

Answers mail and phone inquiries about problems with telephone usage, and helps hearing-aid users acquire compatible phones. (All information provided free.) Quarterly publication, *Out Line,* covers national and local efforts to improve telephone communication for hearing-impaired people.

Sears, Roebuck Local retail or catalog stores

Sells closed-captioned adapters and TV sets with adapters. These devices permit the reception of closed-captioned signals so that people with hearing impairment can read the audio portion of programming at the bottom of their screens. (ABC, CBS, NBC and public television now offer many programs with captioning, identified in local TV program guides.)

Self-Help for Hard of Hearing People
P.O. Box 34889, Washington, DC 20034

National organization with local chapters serves people who are hard of hearing and their families and friends. Promotes advocacy, conducts social and recreational programs, publishes bimonthly magazine, *Shhh.*

Telephone companies Local business offices

Supply information about adaptive equipment to facilitate use of telephones by people with hearing impairments.

U.S. Department of Transportation
National Highway Traffic Safety Board
800 Independence Ave., S.W., Washington, DC 20590 • (202) 382-6600

Distributes free brochure, *Tips on Car Care and Safety for Deaf Drivers.*

DIABETES

American Diabetes Association
2 Park Ave., New York, NY 10016 • (212) 683-7444

This national organization of scientific and medical professionals and volunteers works with diabetics and their families to provide education and support services through local chapters. Publishes excellent bimonthly magazine, *Diabetes Forecast,* and a brochure, *What You Need to Know About Diabetes.*

Diabetes Education Center
4959 Excelsior Blvd., Minneapolis, MN 55416 • (612) 927-3393

Offers a number of educational materials for diabetics, including cookbooks and menu-planning information. Send for descriptive price list.

National Eye Institute
Building 31, Room 6A-32, Bethesda, MD 20205 • (301) 496-5248

Distributes a free twenty-page pamphlet, *Diabetes and Your Eyes.*

HEAD INJURY

National Head Injury Foundation
280 Singletary Lane, Framingham, MA 01701 • (617) 879-7433

National organization serves people who suffer from head injury that has caused brain damage or intellectual or behavioral impairment, and their families. Supplies information about acute and long-term care facilities and rights of the handicapped, offers large variety of support services through local chapters in all parts of country, publishes *National Head Injury Foundation Newsletter* quarterly.

HEART DISEASE AND STROKE

American Heart Association
7320 Greenville Ave., Dallas, TX 75231 • (214) 750-5551

Supports research on the causes, prevention and treatment of heart disease, maintains lists of local Stroke Clubs which provide mutual support for stroke patients and their families, gives information about local services, publishes patient-education materials on heart disease, stroke, heart attack, high blood pressure, angina, heart surgery, pacemakers and nutrition. Contact local chapter for publication list.

High Blood Pressure Information Center
120/80 National Institutes of Health, Bethesda, MD 20205

Distributes free copies of *High Blood Pressure Facts for You and Your Family*, *High Blood Pressure and What You Can Do About It*, and *Watch Your Blood Pressure!*

International Association of Pacemaker Patients
P.O. Box 54305, Atlanta, GA 30308 • (800) 241-6993

Supplies support services to people with pacemakers and to their families. Provides members with a Telephonic EKG and Pacemaker Monitoring Service, as well as medical-alert identification bracelets and necklaces; publishes *Pulse*, an excellent bimonthly magazine for pacemaker wearers. Contact for information about local chapters.

The Mended Hearts
7320 Greenville Ave., Dallas, TX 55231 • (214) 750-5442

Serves heart surgery patients through person-to-person visitation before and after surgery, sponsors local support chapters for patients and their families. List of local chapters available on request.

National Heart, Lung and Blood Institute
Office of Information, Bethesda, MD 20014

Distributes free brochures: *The Human Heart: A Living Pump; A Handbook of Heart Terms; How Doctors Diagnose Heart Disease; Fact Sheet: Arteriosclerosis; Questions About Weight, Salt and High Blood Pressure;* and the Medicine for the Layman series which includes *The Heart; The Brain; Heart Attacks;* and *High Blood Pressure.*

LUNG DISEASE

American Lung Association

1740 Broadway, New York, NY 10019 • (212) 245-8000

Maintains list of pulmonary rehabilitation centers, smoking cessation clinics and national facilities and services; publishes material on emphysema, chronic bronchitis, tuberculosis and other lung diseases (available free to laymen). Local chapters provide information and some direct services. Consult national office or telephone book for nearest chapter.

Emphysema Anonymous

P.O. Box 66, Fort Myers, FL 33902 • (813) 334-4226

This self-help group for persons suffering from emphysema offers personal counselling and support through local chapters; publishes a quarterly newsletter, *Batting the Breeze.* Supported by contributions and a volunteer staff.

LUPUS ERYTHEMATOSUS

Lupus Foundation of America

4434 Covington Highway, Decatur, GA 30035 • (404) 289-7453

Provides information: lists of local chapters, referral lists of physicians experienced in treating lupus, patient-education materials which explain lupus and currently available treatments. Nominal charge for some pamphlets and books; catalog on request.

MENTAL HEALTH

Mental Health Association

1800 North Kent St., Arlington, VA 22209 • (703) 528-6405

Provides information on services, insurance, research, employment, legislation and litigation, rehabilitation and citizen activism to assist persons with mental illness. Extensive publication list includes *Helping the Mental Patient at Home* and *On Understanding Depression.* Contact national office for catalog and information about local chapters and services.

NEUROLOGICAL DISORDERS

American Parkinson's Disease Association

116 John St., New York, NY 10038 • (212) 732-9550

Subsidizes sixteen treatment clinics and maintains a list of self-help groups nationwide. Publishes semiannual newsletter, containing information about research, new treatments, and medications; also *A Manual for Patients With PD; Aids, Equipment and Suggestions to Help in Activities for Daily Living; Speech Problems in PD;* and *Home Exercises for Patients With PD.*

Amyotrophic Lateral Sclerosis Society of America
15300 Ventura Blvd., Suite 315, Sherman Oaks, CA 91403 • (213) 990-2151

Provides information and referral services; through local Muscular Dystrophy chapters, offers financial help and community services. Distributes *Amyotrophic Lateral Sclerosis: Information for Patients and Their Families.*

Association for Alzheimer's and Related Diseases
4141 Parklawn #105, Edina, MN 55435 • (612) 830-1043

Promotes research, help and advocacy for patients with premature senility and their families; sponsors mutual support groups and distributes free literature.

Committee to Combat Huntington's Disease
250 W. 57th St., Suite 2016, New York, NY 10107 • (212) 757-0443

Operates a referral service for diagnostic and treatment centers, genetic counselling and other patient and family needs. Operates a national hot line from 9 A.M. to 5 P.M. weekdays. Distributes a wide variety of educational materials, some free of charge; catalog on request.

Epilepsy Concern
1282 Wynnewood Drive, West Palm Beach, FL 33409 • (305) 967-7616

Helps in starting self-help groups of persons with epilepsy and their families; distributes Epilepsy Concern Starter Kit and a newsletter, Concern.

Epilepsy Foundation of America
4351 Garden City Drive, Landover, MD 20785 • (301) 459-3700

Local chapters provide information and referral services and assistance with individual problems; national office distributes helpful brochures and a listing of books about epilepsy, gives referrals to local chapters.

National Institute of Neurological and Communicative Disorders
National Institutes of Health   Information Office, Bethesda, MD 20205

Publishes a Hope Through Research series: *Cerebral Palsy, Epilepsy, Parkinson's Disease, Multiple Sclerosis, Muscular Dystrophy, Huntington's Disease, Amyotrophic Lateral Sclerosis, Aphasia* and *Spinal Cord Injury.* Also the What You Should Know About series: *Stroke and Stroke Prevention, Brain Tumors and Spinal Cord Tumors, Myasthenia Gravis, Dizziness Including Ménière's Disease* and *Alzheimer's Disease.*

Muscular Dystrophy Association
810 Seventh Ave., New York, NY 10019 • (212) 586-0808

Sponsors research and free medical services for forty neuromuscular diseases at muscular dystrophy clinics nationwide: diagnosis, treatment and genetic and family counselling; sponsors camps and recreational programs and provides other support services to patients and families; distributes free literature and a quarterly magazine for patients, *TIPS.* Local chapters help with purchase or rental of orthopedic aids, drugs and medical transportation.

Myasthenia Gravis Foundation

15 E. 26th St., New York, NY 10010 • (212) 889-8157

Promotes research and education; sponsors MG clinics nationwide and provides drugs at reduced cost. Local chapters provide information and referral, and peer counselling, and sponsor self-help groups. Free publications and information about local chapters and clinics on request.

National Amyotrophic Lateral Sclerosis Foundation

185 Madison Ave., New York, NY 10016 • (212) 679-4016

Sponsors research, patient clinics and numerous local chapters for ALS patients and their families. Distributes *Home Care for the Patient With Amyotrophic Lateral Sclerosis* and other helpful brochures; publishes a newsletter, *National's Update.*

National Huntington's Disease Association

128A E. 74th St., New York, NY 10021 • (212) 744-0302

Supports research to find cause, prevention and cure for Huntington's disease; offers nationwide network of support services, including crisis hot lines, to H.D.-affected patients and their families. Distributes free twelve-page pamphlet, *Huntington's Disease,* and *A Neurologist Speaks With H.D. Families;* publishes a quarterly newsletter, *HD News.*

National Multiple Sclerosis Society

205 E. 42nd St., New York, NY 10017 • (212) 986-3240

Promotes research and services for patients with MS; operates seventy-eight MS clinical centers throughout the country. Local chapters offer information, counselling, referral, medical equipment and many other services. Contact national office for information about local chapters and a price list of helpful publications, including *A Manual on Multiple Sclerosis.*

National Parkinson Foundation

1501 N.W. Ninth Ave., Miami, FL 33136 • (305) 547-6666

Sponsors research and patient services through the Parkinson Rehabilitation and Research Institute of Miami. Provides diagnosis, treatment and rehabilitation services regardless of ability to pay. Distributes two helpful brochures: *What the Patient Should Know About Parkinson's Disease* and *Psychological Factors in the Management of Parkinson's Disease.*

Parkinson's Disease Foundation

William Black Medical Research Building, 640-650 W. 168th St., New York, NY 10032 • (212) 923-4700 or 694-3480

Although primarily a research organization, this foundation offers some patient services, such as free literature, information and referral to Parkinson specialists or self-help groups.

United Cerebral Palsy Association

66 E. 34th St., New York, NY 10016 • (212) 481-6300

Supports research and provides services to patients, including information about programs, clinics and local support chapters.

United Parkinson Foundation

220 South State St., Chicago, IL 60604 • (312) 922-9734

Promotes research and information about Parkinson's disease. Members entitled to use mail-order pharmacy for low-cost prescription drugs. Drug list and educational materials on request; also distributes background literature, exercise instructions and a quarterly newsletter for patient and family education.

SPINAL CORD INJURY

National Spinal Cord Injury Foundation

369 Elliot St., Newton Upper Falls, MA 02164 • (617) 964-0521

Serves paraplegics and quadriplegics by promoting research, improved treatment and advocacy; provides peer counselling for persons with spinal cord injuries and other severe physical disabilities. Publications include *Options: Spinal Cord Injury and the Future, Handbook for Paraplegics and Quadriplegics,* and *How to Be Healthier Through Proper Nutrition.* Price list on request.

Paralyzed Veterans of America

4350 East-West Hwy., Suite 900, Washington, DC 20014 • (301) 652-2135

Serves paralyzed veterans and other disabled people and their families through research, rehabilitation, education, legislative assistance, advocacy, service programs and wheelchair sports programs. Local chapters offer counselling. Publishes *Introduction to Paraplegia, Recreation and Competitive Wheelchair Sports* and a monthly newsletter, *Paraplegic News.* See "Housing and Home Services" in Appendix B for PVA's home modification manuals. Price list on request.

Organizations Providing Specific Types of Services

The resources listed in this appendix relate particularly to Chapter 6, "Getting Back Into the Real World."

PERSONAL CARE: CLOTHING AND LIVING AIDS

Amputee Shoe and Glove Exchange 1635 Warwickshire Drive,
Dr. and Mrs. R. E. Wainerdi Houston, TX 77077

This free service matches amputees who need opposite shoes or gloves. All exchanges of shoes or gloves are between matched amputees.

Care-Sew-Much Designs
1920 Sheely Drive, Ft. Collins, CO 80526 • (303) 482-6590

Sells ready-made adaptive clothing for people of all ages and sexes with special needs. Descriptive flyers, price list and fabric samples available for nominal charge. Specify sex and type of disability.

Fashion Handee for You 7674 Park Ave., Lowville, NY 13367

Offers sewing kits and complete garments for women with physical handicaps. Nominal charge for catalog refundable with first order.

FashionAble   Rocky Hill, NJ 08553 • (609) 921-2563

Offers a wide variety of self-help items, including easy-to-use clothing. Catalog for nominal charge.

Help Yourself Aids   P.O. Box 289, Elmhurst, IL 60126

Sells wheelchair accessories and aids for eating, dressing, recreation, communication and hygiene. Free thirty-page catalog on request.

Iowa State University Cooperative Extension Service
                                             Ames, IA 50010 • (515) 294-4576

Distributes *Clothing to Fit Your Needs*, a thirteen-page booklet suggesting modifications on ready-made garments to accommodate problems related to disability.

Karen Nemeth
       Jacksonville State University, Jacksonville, AL 36101 • (205) 435-9820

Distributes *Undergarments for Those With Special Needs*, an eight-page monograph about making or remodelling undergarments with suggestions about design, fabrics and care.

Kay Caddel   Route 8, Box 12T2, Lubbock, TX 79407

Distributes *Measurements, Guidelines and Solutions*, a manual which describes how to take clothing measurements on a wheelchair-bound or bedridden person and adjust patterns for home sewing.

Michigan State University Cooperative Extension Service
                                     East Lansing, MI 48824 • (517) 355-1855

Distributes a set of bulletins, *Clothes for Independent Living*. Other free bulletins include: *Action Pleats, Clothing Comfort (When Using Crutches), Comfort for Wheelchair Travel, Convenience Fastenings, Lap Robe Skirts* and *Undercover Convenience*.

New Look Patient Apparel   505 Pearl Street, Buffalo, NY 14202

Sells adaptive clothing for people with disabilities. Catalog on request.

Nuday Creations   P.O. Box 7029, Fort Collins, CO 80525

Sells fashionable adaptive clothing for people with handicaps. Catalog on request for nominal charge.

On the Rise   2282 Four Oaks Grange Rd., Eugene, OR 97402

Sells adaptive clothing for people with special needs. Catalog for nominal charge.

PRIDE (Promote Real Independence for the Disabled and Elderly)
             1159 Poquonnock Rd., Groton, CT 06340 • (203) 447-7433

Non-profit organization promotes independence for the handicapped and elderly in home management and personal grooming. Provides modifications and alterations of existing wardrobe, and patterns and designs for customized clothing. Distributes *Dressing With Pride*, a book of sewing instructions for making and adapting clothing.

PTL Designs   Route #2, Box 255, Perkins, OK 74059 • (918) 372-4322

Sells customized clothing for physically handicapped men, women and children through the mail. Garments designed to provide ease, comfort, durability and style. Free catalog and measuring instructions on request.

Ruth Rubin Feldman National Odd Shoe Exchange
          3100 Neilson Way—220, Santa Monica, CA 90405 • (213) 392-4416

Serves persons who need only one shoe or require different shoe sizes for each foot. Acts as clearinghouse for matching people with compatible sizes and tastes. Nominal annual membership fee.

Sears, Roebuck Home Health-Care Catalog   Local retail or catalog stores

This mail-order catalog of home health needs, special garments and incontinence supplies is available from any Sears retail or catalog store.

Sister Kenny Institute
          Publication Department, Abbott-Northwestern Hospital,
          2727 Chicago Ave., Minneapolis, MN 55407 • (612) 874-4175

Publishes *Clothing for the Handicapped: Fashions for Adults and Children.* Send for publications catalog and current price list.

Talon/Velcro
Consumer Education   41 E. 51st St.,
                                                          New York, NY 10022

Distributes *Convenience Clothing and Closures,* which contains hints for clothing selection, information about closures, designs to help with special needs, instructions for garment adaptation and a chart for specific disabilities.

Textile Research Center   P.O. Box 5217, Lubbock, TX 79417

Distributes patterns of clothing and accessories for the physically and mentally handicapped. Free descriptive flyer, *The Natural Creations,* and price list on request.

Vocational Guidance and Rehabilitation Services Sewing Department
          2239 E. 55th St., Cleveland, OH 44103 • (216) 431-7800

Pictorial catalog, *Clothing and Aids for the Physically Disabled,* shows designs and special features of clothing and living aids. Nominal charge.

HOUSING AND HOME SERVICES

Clearinghouse on the Handicapped
Office of Education and Special Rehabilitative Services
          400 Maryland Ave., S.W., Washington, DC 20202 • (202) 245-0080

Responds to inquiries on wide range of topics concerning handicapped, including location of independent living services. All services free of charge.

National HomeCaring Council
          67 Irving Place, New York, NY 10003 • (212) 674-4990

Establishes and maintains standards for homemaker and home health-aide programs, operates information and referral service for those seeking homemakers or home health aides; distributes free materials to guide in selection of safe, efficient and effective in-home services.

Paralyzed Veterans of America
4350 East-West Hwy., Suite 900, Washington, DC 20014 • (301) 652-2135

Publishes helpful manuals on home modification: *Home in a Wheelchair: House Designs for Easier Wheelchair Living; Wheelchair in the Kitchen;* and *Wheelchair Bathrooms.* Price list on request.

Upjohn HealthCare Services
Director of Customer Relations, 3651 Van Rick Drive, Kalamazoo, MI 49002 • (616) 385-6800

Provides at-home health care including skilled nursing; physical, speech and occupational therapy; home health aides; homemakers and medical social services. Medically prescribed services often covered by Medicare, Medicaid or health insurance. Free publication, *Office Directory,* lists local service offices.

U.S. Department of Housing and Urban Development
Office of Independent Living for the Disabled
Room 9106, 541 7th St., Washington, DC 20410 • (202) 755-7366

Provides up-to-date information about housing, rent subsidies and independent living facilities for the handicapped. Distributes free literature: *Changing Environments for People With Disabilities, H.U.D. Programs That Can Help the Handicapped* and *Alternate Housing for the Handicapped.*

Veterans Administration   (see below)

Prepared *Handbook for Design: Specially Adapted Housing* (Pub. 051-000-00125), an eighty-page booklet which provides specific details for adaptive housing designs. Available from Superintendent of Documents, U.S. Government Printing Office, Washington, DC 20402.

EMPLOYMENT AND EDUCATION

Control Data Corporation
Public Affairs, HQS13M, Control Data Corporation, P.O. Box O, Minneapolis, MN 55440

Provides information about local companies offering home employment involving computers.

Goodwill Industries of America   9200 Wisconsin Avenue, N.W., Washington, DC 20814 • (301) 530-6500

Over 175 member organizations offer testing, job-skill training, rehabilitative therapy and counselling to people with physical or mental handicaps. After training, clients are placed in regular work force, or given jobs at home or in sheltered workshops. Local organizations vary in kind and scope of service offered; some provide day nurseries, summer camps or adaptive housing for handicapped and elderly.

Human Resources Center
  I. U. Willets Rd. at Searingtown Rd., Albertson, NY 11507 • (516) 747-5400

Responds to inquiries about employment services for handicapped. Distributes *Vocational and Educational Opportunities for the Disabled* by Anita Tritell, thirty-six-page booklet describing evaluation, training, placement, and counselling in a variety of settings. Write to products manager for Catalog of Publications.

Job Service
Division of U.S. Dept. of Industry, Labor and Human Relations Local office

Operates over two thousand local offices for counselling and placement of people having trouble finding employment. Assists with workers' compensation forms. Referrals to other agencies for testing, on-the-job training and other employment programs. Consult telephone directory for nearest office.

Joseph Bulova School
  40-24 62nd St., Woodside, NY 11377 • (212) 424-2929

Offers watchmaking, watch repair, precision technology and jewelry repair on an individualized basis to handicapped students; also provides some job counselling and placement services. Residential students receive health services, counselling and recreation. Financial aid available to qualifying students. Free brochure on request.

National Home Study Council
  1601 18th St., N.W., Washington, DC 20009 • (202) 234-5100

Distributes free information about home-study programs, including *Directory of Accredited Home Study Schools,* which lists over eighty schools and the courses they provide.

National University Continuing Education Association
  One Dupont Circle, N.W., Washington, DC 20036 • (202) 659-3130

Distributes *Guide to Independent Study Through Correspondence Instruction.* Book lists twelve thousand correspondence courses from approved schools, along with course descriptions, admission requirements, financial costs and aid. Available from Peterson Guides Book Order Department, Box 978, Edison, NJ 08817 and some public libraries.

President's Committee on Employment of the Handicapped
  Office of Publications, 1111 20th Street, N.W.,
  Washington, DC 20210 • (202) 653-5157

Distributes free publications, including *Careers for the Homebound: Home Study Educational Opportunities; Student Consumer's Guide: Six Federal Financial Aid Programs;* and *How to Communicate to and About People Who Happen to Be Handicapped.* Also: *Getting Through College With a Disability: A Summary of Services Available on 500 Campuses for Students With Handicapping Conditions;* and *A Bright Future: Your Guide to Work.*

Small Business Administration
> Office of Public Information, 1441 L Street, N.W.,
> Washington, DC 20005 • (202) 655-4000

Offers assistance to people who want to start their own small business, through low-interest loans, technical assistance, market analysis and other information. Consult telephone directory or write for free literature and information about nearest local office.

RECREATION AND TRAVEL

American Athletic Association of the Deaf
> 3916 Lantern Drive, Silver Spring, MD 20902

Free information on request.

American Automobile Association
Traffic Safety Department
> 8111 Gatehouse Rd., Falls Church, VA 22047 • (703) 222-6671

Distributes free copies of *The Handicapped Driver's Mobility Guide*, a seventy-five page brochure with information about selecting a vehicle, about adaptive driving equipment, modifications to a vehicle and driving schools for disabled persons. Brochure is also available from some local AAA clubs.

American Blind Bowling Association
> 15 N. Bellaire Ave., Louisville, KY 40206 • (502) 896-8039

Free information on request.

American Camping Association
Bradford Woods
> 5040 State Road, 67 North, Martinsville, IN 46151 • (317) 342-8456

Bradford Woods is Indiana University's outdoor education, recreation and camping center. Summer residential programs provide about five hundred campers (ages eight to eighty) with one-to-six-week camping experience. Attracts disabled campers from throughout world. Free information about Bradford Woods and other camping facilities for disabled people is available on request.

American Red Cross
> National Headquarters, 17th St. at D St., N.W.,
> Washington, DC 20006 • (202) 737-8300

Many local chapters of the American Red Cross offer Adapted Aquatics and other programs for people with disabilities. Contact national office or local chapter for details.

American Wheelchair Bowling Association
> 6718 Pinehurst Drive, Evansville, IN 47711 • (812) 867-6503

Free information on request.

American Wheelchair Pilots Association
> 1621 E. 2nd Ave., Mesa, AZ 85204 • (602) 831-4262

Free information on request.

Amtrak
National Railroad Passenger Corp.
400 N. Capitol Street, N.W., Washington, DC 20001 • (800) 523-6591

Offers free copies of *Access Amtrak: A Guide to Amtrak Services for Elderly and Handicapped Travellers.*

Architectural and Transportation Barriers Compliance Board
330 C Street, S.W., Washington, DC 20202 • (202) 245-1591

Distributes free single copies of *Access Travel: Airports—A Guide to Accessibility of Terminals,* which has accessibility tables for major airports in U.S. and other countries.

Avis Rent-a-Car (800) 331-1212

Offers cars equipped with hand controls at most large cities. Requires three weeks' notice. (See also Hertz and National in this listing.)

Blind Outdoor Leisure Development
533 E. Main St., Aspen, CO 81611 • (303) 925-8922

Free information on request.

Continental Trailways 1500 Jackson St., Dallas, TX 75201 • (214) 655-7895

Offers "Good Samaritan Plan" which allows handicapped traveller and companion to travel together for price of single ticket. Their new terminals are barrier-free. For further information contact local terminals or national office.

Disabled Sportsmen of America P.O. Box 26, Vinton, VA 24179

Free information on request.

George Washington University Medical Center
Division of Rehabilitation Medicine, Research and Training Center
2300 I Street, N.W., Suite 714, Washington, DC 20037 • (202) 676-3506

Distributes *Assisting the Wheelchair User* for a nominal charge.

Golden Access Passports (see below)

"Passport"—a lifetime pass—allows holder and other car occupants a 50 percent discount on fees to use federal recreational facilities. Proof of entitlement to federal benefits because of blindness or permanent disability is required. Obtain passport from regional offices of National Park Service, U.S. Forest Service or at entrances to federal parks, forest areas and recreational or historical parks.

Greyhound Lines
Customer Relations, Greyhound Tower, Phoenix, AZ 85077 • (602) 248-5267

Offers "Helping Hand Service" which allows handicapped traveller and companion to travel together for price of single ticket. Wheelchairs carried free. For further information, contact local terminals or national office.

Handy-Cap Horizons
3250 E. Loretta Dr., Indianapolis, IN 46227 • (317) 784-5777

This international travel club, run by volunteers, arranges discounted tours for members who are disabled or want to travel at slow pace. Members receive quarterly magazine and news of upcoming tours.

Health Sports   1455 W. Lake St., Minneapolis, MN 55408

Free information on request.

Hertz Rent-a-Car   (800) 654-3131

Offers cars equipped with hand controls at most large cities. Require ten days' notice. (See also Avis and National in this listing.)

Human Resources Center
I.U. Willets Road, Albertson, NY 11507 • (516) 747-5400

Distributes *Boating for the Handicapped: Guidelines for the Physically Disabled* by Eugene Hedley, which suggests wide range of activities and equipment for recreational boating. Includes list of recreational organizations for handicapped.

Indoor Sports Club
1145 Highland St., Napoleon, OH 43545 • (419) 592-5756

National organization with local chapters and members-at-large promotes social activities, sports and better access for physically disabled people. Publishes bimonthly *National Hookup*. More information on request.

Intermedic   777 Third Ave., New York, NY 10017 • (212) 678-0150

Maintains file of English-speaking physicians from two hundred countries, who are willing to provide emergency care to Intermedic members. Members receive directory of participating physicians and their telephone numbers, immunization information, suggested medications to carry and a personal data form.

International Association for Medical Assistance to Travellers
736 Centre Street, Lewiston, NY 14092 • (716) 754-4883

Offers brochure listing English-speaking doctors in foreign countries who agree to its fee schedules and standards, as well as a Travelers Clinical Record form, World Immunization Chart and Malaria Risk Chart. Requests voluntary contribution. Foundation encourages study of medical aspects of travel and geographical health.

International Committee of Silent Sports
Gallaudet College, 800 Florida Ave., N.E.,
Washington, DC 20002 • (202) 651-5114

Promotes sports for deaf. Free information on request.

Minnesota Outward Bound School
P.O. Box 250, Long Lake, MN 55356 • (612) 473-5476

Offers an Outward Bound outdoor adventure program for the disabled. Free information on request.

**Mobility International
Central Bureau of Educational Visits and Exchanges**
Columbo St., London, ES1 8DP, England

Provides information about travel for physically handicapped persons. Branches situated throughout Europe promote exchanges among handicapped persons from various countries.

**Moss Rehabilitation Hospital
Travel Information Center**
12th Rd. and Tabor Rd., Philadelphia, PA 19141 • (215) 329-5715

Offers free services to hadicapped travellers, including suggestions about where to go, how to get there, where to stay and what to see. Does not make travel arrangements.

Motel chains' and hotel chains' directories for accessible accommodations
(see below)

Many motel and hotel chains offer directories which list accessible accommodations at their various locations. Chains include Best Western, Holiday Inn, Howard Johnson's, Quality Inn, Ramada Inn, TraveLodge, and the Marriott, Hyatt and Sheraton corporations. Travellers should check accessibility details carefully and place reservations well in advance. Call toll-free numbers of these chains to obtain free directories.

National Archery Association
1750 E. Boulder St., Colorado Springs, CO 80909 • (303) 578-4576

Free information on request.

National Car Rental System
(800) 328-4567

Offers cars equipped with hand controls at most large cities. Requires seventy-two hours' notice. (See also Avis and Hertz in this listing.)

National Inconvenienced Sportsman's Association
2215 Allegheny Rd., El Dorado Hills, CA 95630

Free information on request.

National Wheelchair Athletic Association
Templeton Gap Road, Suite C, Colorado Springs, CO 80907 • (303) 632-0698

Promotes wheelchair sports, including archery, various field events, slalom, table tennis, swimming, track, weightlifting and pentathlon. Membership open to wheelchair athletes between ages of thirteen and sixty-five and anyone who wants to promote wheelchair sports. Has over fifteen regional groups and two thousand members nationwide. Sponsors regional events and National Wheelchair Games. National champions compete in international events.

National Wheelchair Softball Association
P.O. Box 737, Sioux Falls, SD 57101

Free information on request.

North American Riding for the Handicapped Association
P.O. Box 100, Ashburn, VA 22011 • (703) 471-1621

Free information on request.

Rehabilitation International U.S.A.
                20 W. 40th St., New York, NY 10018 • (212) 869-9907

Distributes free copies of *International Directory of Access Guides* which
lists guides to fifteen countries in North America and Europe; covers air and
rail travel and wheelchair accessibility to hotels, restaurants and leisure facilities.

Society for the Advancement of Travel for the Handicapped
                26 Court St., Brooklyn, NY 11242 • (212) 858-5483

SATH promotes travel for disabled and acts as clearinghouse for information
about travel agencies to make arrangements for accessible accommodations.

National Park Service
U.S. Department of the Interior   (see below)

Distributes *Access National Parks,* guide to national parks including descriptions of services, accessibility, and medical care for the handicapped and in-
terpretive and special programs for the hearing and visually impaired.
Available from Superintendent of Documents, U.S. Government Printing
Office, Washington, DC 20402.

National Committee on Arts for the Handicapped
        1825 Connecticut Ave., N.W., Washington, DC 20009 • (202) 332-6960

Furthers awareness of arts in handicapped people and encourages development of arts programs for them; provides information resources and technical and research assistance; sponsors Very Special Arts Festivals to
demonstrate and celebrate artistic ability and skill of people with handicaps.

President's Committee on Employment of the Handicapped
        111 20th Street, N.W., Rm. 606, Washington, DC 20036 • (202) 653-5157

Distributes free copies of *Highway Rest Areas for Handicapped Travelers,*
which lists over eight hundred barrier-free highway rest areas on interstate
highways throughout the continental U.S.

U.S. Association of Blind Athletes
        55 W. California Ave., Beach Haven, NJ 08008 • (609) 492-1017

Free information on request.

U.S. Deaf Skiers Association
                2 Sunset Hill Rd., Simsbury, CT 06070 • (203) 244-3070

Free information on request.

Vinland National Center
                3675 Ihduhapi Rd., Loretto, MN 55357 • (612) 479-3555

VNC is health-sports education and training center for disabled. Sponsors
programs at Center and throughout country to encourage active participation in sports to enhance personal well-being, strength and endurance. Free
information on request.

Wheelchair Motorcycle Association
                101 Torrey St., Brockton, MA 02401 • (617) 583-8614

Free information on request.

ADVOCACY

American Coalition of Citizens With Disabilities
1200 15th St., N.W., Suite 201, Washington, DC 20005 • (202) 785-4265

Promotes research, education and advocacy on behalf of the legal rights of disabled people; provides information and referral services regarding specific problems. Publishes a number of helpful books and brochures on advocacy techniques; descriptive price list on request.

American Council of the Blind   1211 Connecticut Ave., N.W., Suite 506, Washington, DC 20036 • (202) 833-1251

Offers free, direct legal assistance to groups in discrimination and benefits cases and to individuals in precedent cases. Distributes information on many services for the blind and a monthly magazine which updates developments in legislation, education and employment for the blind. Available in large print or braille, on disc or cassette.

Center for Legal Advocacy
Legal Center for Handicapped Citizens
1060 Bannock St., Suite 316, Denver, CO 80204
• (303) 573-0542 or (800) 332-6356 (Colorado only)

Offers advocacy and legal service to disabled persons who encounter discrimination in education, employment, housing or social services. Promotes education and legislative programs for legal rights of the disabled.

Center on Human Policy   216 Ostrom Ave., Syracuse, NY 13210
Syracuse University   • (315) 423-3851

Promotes legal rights of people with disabilities for integrated educational, vocational, rehabilitative and residential services. Free advice and backup assistance to individual consumers and advocacy groups. Provides consumers with information regarding legal rights and strategies for change. Free catalog of publications on request.

Disability Rights Center   1346 Connecticut Ave., N.W., Suite 1124, Washington, DC 20036 • (202) 223-3304

Primarily concerned with enforcing legal rights of federal employees, it offers a number of publications that deal with this issue. Publications include *Medical Devices and Equipment for the Disabled* and *Consumer Warranty Law: Your Rights and How to Enforce Them*. Descriptive price list available

Legal Services Corporation
733 15th St., N.W., Washington, DC 20005 • (202) 272-4000

Established by Congress to support legal services for the poor. Assists disabled individuals who meet financial eligibility guidelines with legal problems through approximately 355 neighborhood offices.

Mental Health Law Project
2021 L St., N.W., Suite 800, Washington, DC 20036 • (202) 467-5730

Offers legal advice and assistance to people with mental and emotional disorders or developmental disabilities who are denied their legal rights.

National Association for Hearing and Speech Action
10801 Rockville Pike, Rockville, MD 20852 • (301) 897-8682

NAHSA is a consumer advocacy affiliate of the American Speech-Language-Hearing Association. Assists with legal and other problems related to communication disorders, maintains listing of professionally accredited clinical service programs in each state. For information call collect weekdays 8 A.M.–4:30 P.M.

National Association of the Physically Handicapped
76 Elm St., London, OH 43140

A self-help action group which promotes the social, economic and physical welfare of the physically handicapped. Most local chapters located in Eastern U.S., but anyone can join as a member-at-large. Has annual national convention and publishes quarterly newsletter. Free descriptive literature on request.

National Center for Law and the Deaf
7th St. and Florida Ave., N.E., Washington, DC 20002 • (202) 651-5454

Provides a variety of legal services to the deaf community, including representation, counselling, information and education. Operates legal services clinic for Washington, D.C. residents. Publishes quarterly newsletter and educational brochures on a variety of subjects.

President's Committee on Employment of the Handicapped
1111 20th St., N.W., 6th Floor, Washington, DC 20036 • (202) 653-5044

Provides information and publications on employment, architectural accessibility and education, including a *Community Action Guide for Disabled Americans*. Other free brochures include: *Affirmative Action for Disabled People, Affirmative Action to Employ Handicapped People, Affirmative Action to Employ Disabled Veterans and Veterans of the Vietnam Era.*

U.S. Department of Health and Human Services
Public Affairs
Office of Civil Rights
Washington, DC 20201

Distributes free brochure, *Your Rights as a Disabled Person*, which outlines federal regulations against discrimination towards the handicapped.

CHAPTER 1:
"THIS COULDN'T HAPPEN TO ME!": ADJUSTING TO DISABILITY

1. National Safety Council, *Accident Facts* (Washington, D.C.: NSC, 1978); U.S. Bureau of the Census, *Statistical Abstract of the United States: 1982–83* (Washington, D.C.: Government Printing Office, 1982).
2. R. William English, "Correlates of Stigma Towards Physically Disabled Persons," in *Social and Psychological Aspects of Disability: A Handbook for Practitioners*, ed. Joseph Stubbins (Baltimore: University Park Press, 1977), pp. 207–24.
3. Nancy Kerr (Cohn), "Understanding the Process of Adjustment to Disability," ibid., pp. 317–24.
4. Tim Caywood, "A Quadriplegic Young Man Looks At Treatment," ibid., pp. 61–68.
5. Glorya Hale, ed., *The Source Book for the Disabled* (New York and London: Paddington Press, 1979), pp. 8–9 (New York: Holt, Rinehart & Winston, 1982; Bantam, 1983).
6. Interview with Norman Cousins. *See also* his *Anatomy of an Illness: As Perceived by the Patient* (New York: W. W. Norton, 1979; Bantam, 1981).

CHAPTER 2: THE INS AND OUTS OF HOSPITALS

1. Donald S. Kornfield, "The Hospital Environment: Its Impact on the Patient," *Advances in Psychosomatic Medicine*, vol. 8 (1972): pp. 252–70.
2. Lawrence E. Schlesinger, "Staff Authority and Patient Participation in Rehabilitation," in *Social and Psychological Aspects of Disability*, ed. Stubbins, pp. 167–71.

3. Lee Meyerson, article in *Rehabilitation Counseling Bulletin*, vol. 14 (1970): pp. 85–94.
4. Arthur Levin, *Talk Back to Your Doctor: How to Demand and Recognize High Quality Health Care* (Garden City, N.Y.: Doubleday, 1975), pp. 124–26.
5. American Hospital Association, *Hospitals*, vol. 52, no. 22 (November 16, 1978): p. 112.
6. Hilda P. Versluys, "Physical Rehabilitation and Family Dynamics," *Rehabilitation Literature*, vol. 41, no. 3–4 (March–April 1980), pp. 58–65.
7. Irvin G. Wilmot, quoted in "Family Care for Patients to Be Tested," *American Medical News*, April 6, 1979; other information from Wilmot, letter to author.

CHAPTER 3: REHABILITATION ALTERNATIVES

1. Beatrice A. Wright, "Issues in Overcoming Emotional Barriers to Adjustment in the Handicapped," *Rehabilitation Counseling Bulletin*, vol. 11 (1967): pp. 53–59.
2. Versluys, "Physical Rehabilitation," *Rehabilitation Literature*.
3. Ross Mullner et al., "Inpatient Medical Rehabilitation: 1979 Survey of Hospitals and Units" (report by staff of American Hospital Association Data Center).
4. Carroll M. Brodsky and Robert T. Platt, *The Rehabilitation Environment* (Lexington, Mass.: D. C. Heath, Lexington Books, 1978), pp. 13–39.
5. James A. Bitter, "Some Viable Service Delivery Approaches in Rural Rehabilitation," *Rehabilitation Literature*, vol. 33, no. 12 (1972): 354–57.
6. Brodsky and Platt, *Rehabilitation Environment*, p. 68.
7. Ibid., pp. 5–6.
8. I. J. Rossman and Doris R. Schwartz, *The Family Handbook of Home Nursing and Medical Care* (New York: M. Evans, 1968), chapter 7.
9. Levin, *Talk Back to Your Doctor*, p. 155; John J. Regan, "When Nursing Home Patients Complain: The Ombudsman or the Patient Advocate," *The Georgetown Law Journal*, vol. 65-691 (1977): pp. 691–738, N.B. pp. 694 and 735.
10. National Citizens' Coalition for Nursing Home Reform, *Manual*, Secs. I, II and IV; U.S. Dept. of Health, Education and Welfare, Office of Human Development Services, Administration on Aging, *Program Development Handbook for State and Area Agencies on Nursing Home Ombudsman Services for the Elderly*, Washington, D.C., October 1977 (DHEW Pub. No. [OHDS] 78-20022), Chaps. I–III.
11. Geraldine Widmer, Roberta Brill and Adele Schlosser, "Home Health Care: Services and Costs," *Nursing Outlook*, vol. 26, no. 8 (1978): pp. 488–93.

CHAPTER 4: PUTTING CONVALESCENT TIME TO WORK

1. V. A. Christopherson, "The Patient and the Family," *Rehabilitation Literature*, vol. 23, no. 2 (1962): pp. 34–41.
2. M. L. Walker, R. Clark and H. Sawyer, "Sexual Rehabilitation of the

Spinal-Cord Injured: A Program for Counselor Education," *Rehabilitation Counseling Bulletin,* June 1975, p. 281.
3. Mary D. Romano, "Sexuality and the Disabled Female," *Accent on Living,* Winter 1973.
4. Chris Papadopoulos, "How Wives Feel About Coitus After Husband's Heart Attack," *Medical Aspects of Human Sexuality,* vol. 14, no. 8 (1980): pp. 57, 59, 66, 71.
5. Roberta B. Trieschman, "Sexual Dysfunctions Associated with Physical Disabilities," *Archives of Physical Medicine and Rehabilitation,* vol. 56 (1975): pp. 8–13.
6. Theodore M. Cole and Sandra S. Cole, "The Handicapped and Sexual Health," *SIECUS Report,* vol. 4, no. 5 (1976): pp. 1–2, 9–10.
7. Linda Murray, "What Are Medical Students Learning About Sexual Medicine? Not Enough, Says Dr. Harold I. Lief," *Sexual Medicine Today,* Jan. 14, 1981, pp. 6–13.
8. Theodore M. Cole and Dorothea D. Glass, "Sexuality and Physical Disability," *Archives of Physical Medicine and Rehabilitation,* vol. 58, no. 12 (1977): pp. 585–86.
9. Theodore M. Cole, "Sexuality and Physical Disabilities," *Archives of Sexual Behavior,* vol. 4, no. 4 (1975): pp. 389–403.
10. Joseph D. Waxberg and Stella Mostel, "Sex and the Terminally Ill: Overcoming Obstacles to Gratification," *Sexual Medicine Today,* Nov. 1980, pp. 25, 26, 39–40.
11. Adeline M. Hoffman, *Clothing for the Handicapped, the Aged, and Other People With Special Needs* (Springfield, Ill.: Charles C. Thomas, 1979), chapter 5.
12. Beatrice A. Wright, *Physical Disability: A Psychological Approach* (New York: Harper and Row, 1960), pp. 223–37.
13. Ibid., pp. 208–23.

CHAPTER 5: HELP FOR THE HELPERS

1. Thomas H. Holmes and Minoru Masuda, "Psychosomatic Syndrome," *Psychology Today,* vol. 4, no. 3 (1972).
2. John G. Bruhn, "Effects of Chronic Illness on the Family," *The Journal of Family Practice,* vol. 4, no. 6 (1977): 1057–60.
3. Rollo May, *The Meaning of Anxiety* (New York: W. W. Norton, 1977), p. 377.
4. Frederic F. Flack, *Choices: Coping Creatively With Personal Change* (Philadelphia: J. B. Lippincott, 1977), pp. 47, 77.
5. Ibid., p. 80.
6. Hilda P. Versluys, "Physical Rehabilitation and Family Dynamics," *Rehabilitation Literature,* vol. 41, no. 3–4 (March–April 1980), pp. 58–65.
7. Reinhold Niebuhr, "The Serenity Prayer," 1943.

CHAPTER 6: GETTING BACK INTO THE REAL WORLD

1. Arno B. Zimmer, *Employing the Handicapped: A Practical Compliance Manual* (New York: AMACOM, division of American Management Associations, 1981), pp. 219, 229.

2. L. Anthony Magliozzi, personal interview with author, Boston, May 1982.
3. Frank Bowe, *Handicapping America: Barriers to Disabled People* (New York: Harper and Row, 1978), p. 28.
4. Zimmer, *Employing the Handicapped*, p. 30.
5. Kenneth Kolpan, personal interview with author, Boston, May 1982.

CHAPTER 7: "HOW CAN WE PAY FOR ALL THIS?"

1. Don A. Olson, in *Proceedings of the National Training Institute: The Industrially Injured, 1976* (mimeographed report distributed to participants at institute, coordinated by Rehabilitation Institute of Chicago), p. 1.
2. Health Insurance Institute, *Source Book of Health Insurance Data, 1979–80* (Washington, D.C.: H.I.I., 1980), p. 7.
3. Susan Dower (Health Insurance Institute, Washington, D.C.), letter to author, Oct. 28, 1980.
4. Roger M. Pierce (managing editor, *The John Liner Letter*, Wellesley, Mass.), letter to author, Sept. 10, 1980.
5. *Marquette Law Review*, vol. 52 (1969–70): pp. 452–54.
6. INA MEND Institute, *Financial Assistance for the Disabled* (Albertson, N.Y.: INA MEND Inst., Human Resources Center, 1975), p. 12.
7. U.S. Department of Transportation, *Economic Consequences of Automobile Accident Injuries*, a report of the Westat Research Corp., vol. 1 (Washington, D.C.: GPO, 1970).
8. Fred L. Bardenwerper (Defense Research Institute, Inc., Milwaukee, Wis.), letter to author, Sept. 9, 1980.
9. INA MEND Inst., *Financial Assistance*, pp. 12–14.
10. Patrick Magarick, "Some Further Comments on Advance Payments," *Insurance Adjuster*, Oct. 1972.
11. Secretary Volpe quoted in Jeffrey O'Connell, *The Injury Industry and the Remedy of No-Fault Insurance* (Chicago: University of Illinois Press, 1971), p. 181.
12. Roy E. Holloway, "Rehabilitation and the Adjuster," *Canadian Insurance*, vol. 85, no. 6 (1980): pp. 20–22, 60–65.
13. Aaron J. Broder and Vincent J. Mangano III, "Structured Settlements: Insurance Gimmick or Valuable Tool for Injured Plaintiffs?" parts 1, 2, *The National Underwriter*, Aug. 29, 1980, pp. 25–26, 32; Sept. 5, 1980, pp. 31, 38–39. Roger C. Henderson, "Calculating Damages: Economic Uncertainties Point Out the Necessity for Periodic Payments," *Business Insurance*, Sept. 8, 1980, p. 24.
14. W. E. Sedgwick and William C. Judge, "The Use of Annuities in Settlement of Personal Injury Cases," *Insurance Counsel Journal*, Oct. 1974, pp. 584–92.
15. Fred Bardenwerper, letter.
16. Frank Bowe, *Handicapping America: Barriers to Disabled People* (New York: Harper and Row, 1978), p. 24.
17. William G. Johnson, "Income Support and Social Insurance," in *Disability Policies and Government Programs*, ed. Edward D. Berkwitz (New York: Praeger, 1979), p. 17.
18. U.S. Department of Health and Human Services, *Work Disability in the United States*, Social Security Administration Pub. No. 13-11978, Dec. 1980, p. 17.

19. *Milwaukee Journal*, May 9, 1982 (New York Times Service).
20. *Proceedings, National Training Institute*, p. 9.
21. U.S. Chamber of Commerce, *Analysis of Workers' Compensation Laws, 1982*, pp. 15–17.
22. Donald E. Falvin, in *Proceedings, Natl. Training Institute*, p. 37.
23. George P. Sawyer, ibid., p. 27.
24. Bowe, *Handicapping America*, p. 28.
25. Constantina Safilios-Rothschild, *The Sociology and Social Psychology of Disability and Rehabilitation* (New York: Random House, 1970), p. 29.
26. *Proceedings, Natl. Training Institute*, p. 19.
27. Falvin, ibid., p. 37.
28. Ronald Conley, "Should We Break Up Workers' Compensation?" in *Disability Policies and Government Programs*, pp. 168–74.
29. U.S. Dept. of Labor report quoted in *Milwaukee Journal*, July 13, 1980 (Washington Post Service).
30. Lawrence Smedley, in *Proceedings, Natl. Training Institute*, p. 18.
31. Eleanor M. Ross, in ibid., p. 51.
32. Daniel G. Baldyga, *How to Settle Your Own Insurance Claim* (New York: Macmillan, 1968), pp. 110–12.
33. Ibid., p. 113.

Anderson, Vincent. *Exercises and Selfcare Activities for Quadriplegic People.* Bloomington, Ill.: Accent Publications.

This valuable guide for patients and their caregivers offers an exercise program to increase self-sufficiency. Illustrated. (Order from publisher: Box 700, Bloomington IL 61701. Price includes shipping charge.)

Annand, Douglass R., ed. Revised ed. *The Wheelchair Traveler.* Annand Ent., 1979.

This 228-page book lists 6,000 wheelchair-accessible hotels, motels, restaurants and tourist attractions across the United States, Canada, Mexico and Puerto Rico. (Paperback; available from author at Ball Hill Road, Milford NH 03055, and from Accent Special Publications, Box 700, Bloomington IL 61701).

Annas, George J. *The Rights of Hospital Patients.* New York: Avon, 1975

This American Civil Liberties Union handbook explains the rights of hospital patients in easy-to-understand terms. (Paperback.)

Becker, Elle F. *Female Sexuality Following Spinal Cord Injury.* Bloomington, Ill.: Accent Publications.

Excellent resource for women, their spouses and families, and health professionals. Offers many practical suggestions. (Order from publisher: Box 700, Bloomington IL 61701. Price includes shipping charge.)

Belsky, Marvin, and Gross, Leonard. *How to Choose and Use Your Doctor.* Revised ed. New York: Arbor House, 1979.

Offers some good suggestions for improving communication with doctors and obtaining better care from them. (Paperback.)

Bergman, Sue. *Sexuality and the Spinal Cord Injured Woman.* Minneapolis, Minn.: Sister Kenny Institute, 1975.

Suggests sexual possibilities available to women with spinal cord injury, as well as ways to improve communication with sexual partner. (Order from publisher: 800 E. 28th St., Minneapolis, MN 55407.)

Bowe, Frank. *Handicapping America: Barriers to Disabled People.* New York: Harper and Row, 1978.

Details the problems of discrimination that disabled people face in this country, and offers suggestions for improving their circumstances.

Bowe, Frank. *Rehabilitating America: Toward Independence for Disabled and Elderly People.* New York: Harper and Row, 1980.

Author argues for more federal spending on rehabilitation programs and for the removal of barriers. Good background preparation for anyone interested in promoting the integration of disabled people into community life.

Bruck, Lilly. *Access: The Guide to a Better Life for Disabled Americans.* New York: Random House, 1978.

Gives information about employment rights, education, travel, housing, insurance, government services and consumer services—where to write, how to get action and where to find needed resources. (Out of print, but available from public libraries.)

Cary, Jane R. *How to Create Interiors for the Disabled.* New York: Pantheon, 1978.

This excellent book tells how to modify a home for a disabled person and how family can be involved in the rehabilitation process. Lists sources of equipment and other useful information.

Cousins, Norman. *Anatomy of an Illness; As Perceived by the Patient.* New York: W. W. Norton, 1979; Bantam, 1981.

The author describes his own battle with disease and his victory through humor. This widely read book offers excellent advice for combatting the stress of illness.

Dorros, Sidney. *Parkinson's: A Patient's View.* Washington, D.C.: Seven Locks Press, 1981.

A Parkinson's disease patient tells how he achieved accommodation to his disease without surrender. Offers tips on coping, and gives information about treatment centers, local support groups, books and other resources.

Ford, Jack R., et al. *Physical Management for the Quadriplegic Patient.* Philadelphia: F. A. Davis, 1974.

An illustrated guide for assisting quadriplegics with daily living activities. Detailed step-by-step instructions for dressing, grooming and so on. (Out of print, but available from public libraries.)

Galbreaith, Patricia. *What You Can Do for Yourself: Hints for the Handicapped.* New York: Drake, 1974.

Offers many good suggestions for women who must use a wheelchair. (Out of print, but available from public libraries.)

Gollay, Elinor, et al. *The College Guide for Students With Disabilities.* Cambridge, Mass.: ABT Publications, 1976.

This library reference book contains information on college admission testing, financial aid, learning-aid resources, course descriptions, architectural accessibility and legal rights of students.

Gregory, M. F. *Sexual Adjustment: A Guide for the Spinal Cord Injured.* Bloomington, Ill.: Accent Publications, 1974.

Written mainly about sexual adjustment for male paraplegics, but offers important information to individuals with other physical disabilities. (Paperback; order from publisher: Box 700, Bloomington IL 61701.)

Hale, Glorya, ed. *The Source Book for the Disabled.* New York and London: Paddington Press, 1979; New York: Holt, Rinehart & Winston, 1982; Bantam, 1983.

This illustrated guide to easier, more independent living for physically disabled people offers information about all aspects of daily life. An excellent resource for disabled people and their families.

Hoffman, Adeline M. *Clothing for the Handicapped, the Aged, and Other People With Special Needs.* Springfield, Ill.: Charles C. Thomas, 1979.

This comprehensive book about adaptive clothing is an excellent resource.

Hull, Kent. *The Rights of Physically Handicapped People.* New York: Avon, 1979.

Although at times quite technical, this American Civil Liberties Union Handbook is an excellent resource for anyone who wants to fight discrimination of the handicapped. Contains a detailed description of the Rehabilitation Act. (Paperback.)

Katz, Alfred, and Martin, Knute. *A Handbook of Services for the Handicapped.* Westport, Conn. Greenwood Press, 1982.

A reference book of physical-care services, housing, financial aid, employment, vocational rehabilitation, personal and family counselling, services for children and recreation and social activities, with an appendix of service agencies.

Kernaleguen, Anne. *Clothing Designs for the Handicapped.* Forest Grove, Ore.: Hydra Book Co., 1978.

This comprehensive book provides designs for men, women and children. Easy-to-follow directions and illustrations. (Spiral-bound paperback; order from Accent Publications, Box 700, Bloomington IL 61701.)

Klinger, J. R., et al. *Mealtime Manual for the Aged and Handicapped.* New York: Simon and Schuster, 1970.

Prepared by staff of the Institute of Rehabilitative Medicine at NYU Medical Center, this book describes adaptive techniques and devices to deal with food preparation and eating problems. (Out of print, but available from public libraries.)

Kreisler, Nancy, and Kreisler, Jack. *Catalog of Aids for the Disabled.* New York: McGraw-Hill, 1982.

Illustrates aids for the disabled in personal care, dressing, meal preparation, eating, various other household activities, getting around, communication, recreation, travel, accident prevention at home and safety from crime. Lists sources and approximate costs.

Larson, Maren R., et al. *Attendant Care Manual.* Bloomington, Ill.: Accent Publications.

Book describes types of disabilities and the special needs they create, with emphasis on spinal cord injuries. Includes procedures for daily living and first aid, and a daily checklist for attendants. (Spiral-bound paperback; order from publisher: Box 700, Bloomington IL 61701.)

Laurie, Gini. *Housing and Home Services for the Disabled.* Rev. ed. (1st ed. 1977.) Hagerstown, Md.: Harper and Row, 1982.

This book by the editor and publisher of *Rehabilitation Gazette* includes a great variety of information about all aspects of independent living.

Lunt, Suzanne. *A Handbook for the Disabled: Ideas and Inventions for Easier Living.* New York: Charles Scribner's Sons, 1982.

Offers suggestions for daily living, personal care, communication, travel, recreation, and financial help.

May, E. E., et al. *Independent Living for the Handicapped and the Elderly.* Boston: Houghton Mifflin, 1974.

This do-it-yourself book explains techniques and equipment that help with activities of daily living. Contains sources for adaptive clothing and appliances.

Mooney, T., et al. *Sexual Options for Paraplegics and Quadriplegics.* Boston: Little, Brown, 1975.

This excellent book offers many valuable suggestions for people with spinal cord injuries.

Nierenberg, Judith. *A Complete Guide to Understanding and Participating in Your Own Care*. New York: Bobbs-Merrill, 1978.

This book for hospital patients discusses hospital procedures, special units and services, frequently used abbreviations and terms, and diagnostic tests and procedures.

Prichard, Elizabeth, et al. *Home Care: Living With the Dying*. New York: Columbia University Press, 1979.

Although this book chiefly addresses paraprofessionals working with dying patients and their families, it offers many suggestions that families would find helpful.

Reamy, Lois. *TravelAbility*. New York: Macmillan, 1979.

This excellent travel guide tells how to plan a trip, use transportation services and find accessible sites and accommodations throughout the U.S.

Robinault, I. P. *Functional Aids for the Multiply Handicapped*. Hagerstown, Md.: Harper Medical Books, 1973.

Describes functional aids and equipment for general mobility, travel, personal care, communication, learning and recreation.

Rossman, I. J., and Schwartz, Doris R. *The Family Handbook of Home Nursing and Medical Care*. New York: M. Evans, 1968.

This is a good basic book on home nursing techniques, with excellent information. (Out of print, but still available from many public libraries.)

Sarno, J., and Sarno, M. *Stroke: A Guide for Patients and Their Families*. New York: McGraw-Hill, 1979.

This book offers comprehensive information about strokes, and is an excellent resource for families of stroke patients. (Paperback.)

Schellen, K., et al. *Not Made of Stone: The Sexual Problems of Handicapped People*. Springfield, Ill.: Charles C. Thomas, 1974.

A good book for disabled persons, their partners and family members. (Out of print, but available from many public libraries.)

Shaul, S., et al. *Toward Intimacy: Family Planning and Sex Concerns of Physically Disabled Women*. New York: Human Sciences Press, 1978.

Discusses sexual needs of disabled women and offers frank, helpful suggestions. Primary emphasis on women with spinal cord injuries, but suggestions are applicable to any disabled woman. (Paperback.)

Stolten, Jane H. *Home Care: A Guide to Family Nursing*. Boston: Little, Brown, 1975.

An excellent resource book about all aspects of home nursing care, with many illustrations.

Velleman, Ruth A. *Serving Physically Disabled People: An Information Handbook for All Libraries.* New York: R. R. Bowker, 1979.

This library reference book contains extensive listings of publications and services for the handicapped.

Weiss, Louise. *Access to the World: A Travel Guide for the Handicapped.* New York: Chatham Square Press, 1977.

Describes accessible hotels, health facilities, travel agencies and organizations serving disabled people throughout the world. Has a list of access guides to countries and major cities. Also available from the author: 154 E. 29th St., New York, NY 10016.

Zimmer, Arno B. *Employing the Handicapped: A Practical Compliance Manual.* New York: AMACOM, 1981.

This is an excellent book for employers, because it outlines their obligations to disabled employees or job applicants. Also a useful tool for handicapped people who suffer from employment discrimination.

362.4
COO   Coombs, Jan
        Living with the disabled:

DATE DUE		
OCT 29		
APR 0 5 1989		